WALKING PORTLAND

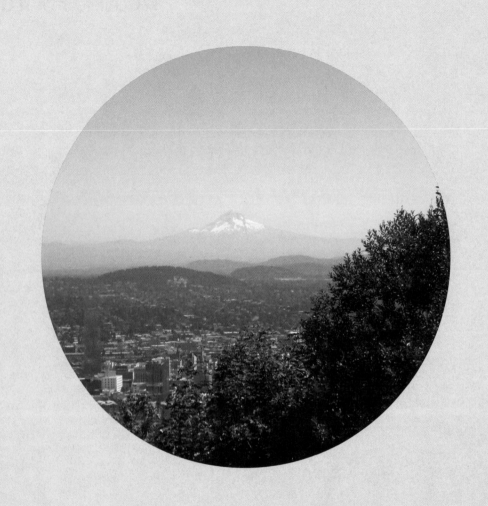

WALKING PORTLAND

30 Tours of Stumptown's Funky Neighborhoods, Historic Landmarks, Parks, Farmers' Markets, and Brewpubs

Becky Ohlsen

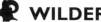 **WILDERNESS PRESS** . . . *on the trail since 1967*

Walking Portland: 30 tours of Stumptown's funky neighborhoods, historic landmarks, parks, farmers' markets, and brewpubs

1st EDITION 2013
    4th printing 2016

Front-cover photos copyright © by Becky Ohlsen except as noted below
Interior photos by Becky Ohlsen except as noted on-page
Maps: Scott McGrew
Cover and book design: Larry B. Van Dyke and Lisa Pletka
ISBN 978-0-89997-681-5; eISBN 978-0-89997-682-2

Manufactured in the United States of America

Published by: **WILDERNESS PRESS**
                AdventureKEEN
                2204 First Avenue South, Suite 102
                Birmingham, AL 35233
                800-443-7227; fax 205-326-1012
                info@wildernesspress.com
                wildernesspress.com

Visit our website for a complete listing of our books, and for ordering information.

Distributed by Publishers Group West

Cover photos: *Front, clockwise from upper right:* Portland Oregon Stag Sign, Old Town (© Daniel Deitschel); Chinatown Gate, Chinatown; Pioneer Courthouse Square, Downtown Park Blocks; The Rare Book Room at Powell's City of Books, Pearl District (© Paul Gerald); Fifteenth Avenue Hophouse, Irvington; Hawthorne Bridge (© Jerry Koch); rose from International Rose Test Garden, Washington Park (© Paul Gerald). *Back, top to bottom: Portlandia* statue, Downtown Park Blocks; Pittock Mansion, Forest Park (© Paul Gerald); International Rose Test Garden, Washington Park.

Frontispiece: View of Mt. Hood

SAFETY NOTICE: Although Wilderness Press and the author have made every attempt to ensure that the information in this book is accurate at press time, they are not responsible for any loss, damage, injury, or inconvenience that may occur to anyone while using this book. You are responsible for your own safety and health while following the walking trips described here. Always check local conditions, know your limitations, and consult a map.

acknowledgments

First off, thanks to Molly Merkle and Holly Cross at Wilderness Press headquarters for their patience in getting this book together, eventually. Also to fellow walking-guide author and erstwhile Portlander Ryan Ver Berkmoes, who roped me into this project in its early stages and made me realize how much I liked the idea of exploring my own city rather than yet another far-flung locale, for a change. I had a lot of help along the way, too, including from Zac Christensen, who hooked me up with Metro trails coordinator Mel Huie; and from Patrick Leyshock, Kate McLaughlin, Zach and Ashton Hull, Mike Russell, DK Holm, and Margo DeBeir, all of whom provided massive amounts of support, intel, and occasionally even dinner.

author's note

Portland's a great town for walking, especially if you aren't the type who melts in rain. The city is mostly flat, the blocks are much shorter than the usual length (which is really only a help for the ego, but still), and there are gorgeous parks and green spaces blanketing every section of the city. (And it's true what they say about April showers—the flowers here in spring are unbelievable.) If you really aren't the Gene Kelly type, you'll find warm and cozy brewpubs, dive bars, coffee shops, and tea houses to duck into on every block; we've recommended several we like for just such circumstances.

Some of the routes here are slightly hilly, and some include unpaved trails through the city's urban forest, so do be prepared and choose your footwear wisely. But Portland has yet another advantage as a walker's paradise: its public transportation system is excellent, so if you wear yourself out, it's usually easy to catch a bus back toward the center of town from most anywhere.

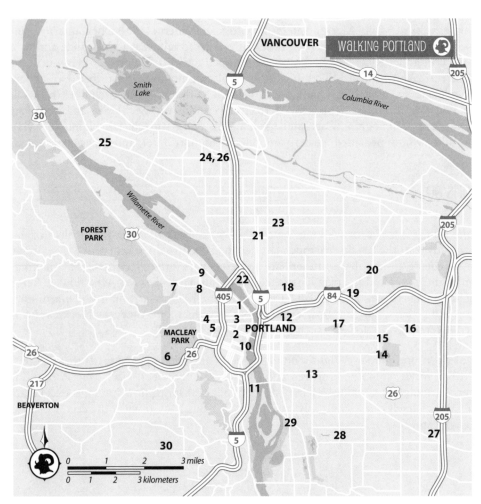

VANCOUVER

WALKING PORTLAND

Smith Lake

Columbia River

25

24, 26

FOREST PARK

Willamette River

23

21

9

7   8

22

18

20

405

5

84   19

1

3   12

4   PORTLAND

5

2   10

17

16

15

14

MACLEAY PARK

6   26

13

11

26

BEAVERTON

29

28

27

30

5

0   1   2   3 miles
0   1   2   3 kilometers

NUMBERS ON THIS LOCATOR MAP CORRESPOND TO WALK NUMBERS.

Table of Contents

INTRODUCTION

Thanks to IFC's hit TV show *Portlandia,* walking might not be the first thing you associate with Portland. In fact, it's probably well down the list, after pedigreed chickens, disapproving lesbian bookstore clerks, *Star Trek* reenactments, and unicycling bagpipers. These days, the familiar slogan "Keep Portland Weird" is more of a description than a call to action: it's simply what we do here.

But part of what keeps Portland so wonderfully weird is also what makes it a brilliant city for walking: a compact, almost European-style layout, with a focus on parks and open spaces—the result of the city's unconventional approach to planning and transportation. Portland is filled with odd little nooks and crannies where locals (and in-the-know visitors) have room to hang out, relax, and explore ideas like "What if we used bicycles to transport our brewpub around the city," or "How about we put a hotel in that crumbling warehouse?"

A walk in Portland thus includes an element of surprise. On any given stroll, you might round a corner to find a pop-up shop selling vintage paperbacks or gluten-free cupcakes shaped like the mayor, for example, and beyond that a manicured Victorian house restored with heartbreaking care. And it may turn out that the beautiful Victorian house is also a coffee shop or a brewpub or both, and so you settle in with your book or cupcake for a pause in its rhododendron-filled back garden.

Granted, for three-fourths of the year this scenario might have a backdrop of rain. Portland is known for its soggy weather, though it's reliably fair and warm in July and August. And all that rain produces some of the most glorious gardens and parks in the country—even ordinary houses in many neighborhoods boast front yards that are landscaping wonders.

The walks we've laid out are neighborhood-focused, so you'll get a flavor of quite a few different parts of town. We've built the routes around places you can duck in for shelter or sustenance if need be. So grab your umbrella and enjoy!

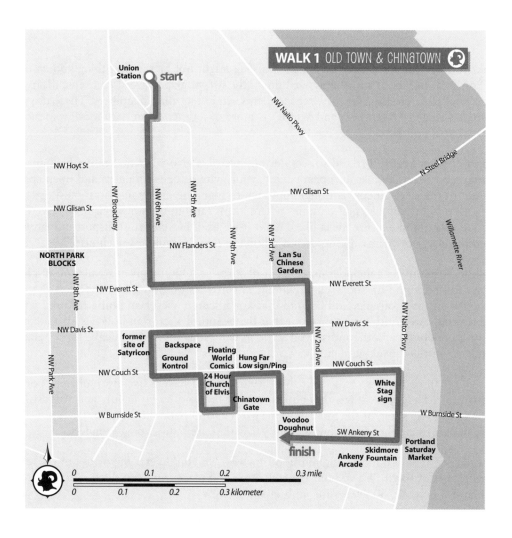

WALK 1 OLD TOWN & CHINaTOWN

Union Station ○ start

NW Naito Pkwy

N Steel Bridge

NW Hoyt St

NW Glisan St

NW Broadway

NW 6th Ave

NW 5th Ave

NW Glisan St

Willamette River

NW Glisan St

NW Flanders St

NW 4th Ave

NW 3rd Ave

Lan Su Chinese Garden

NORTH PARK BLOCKS

NW 8th Ave

NW Everett St

NW Everett St

NW Davis St

NW Davis St

NW Naito Pkwy

former site of Satyricon

Backspace

Floating World Comics

Hung Far Low sign/Ping

NW 2nd Ave

NW Park Ave

Ground Kontrol

NW Couch St

24 Hour Church of Elvis

NW Couch St

White Stag sign

W Burnside St

Chinatown Gate

W Burnside St

Voodoo Doughnut

finish

SW Ankeny St

Ankeny Arcade

Skidmore Fountain

Portland Saturday Market

0   0.1   0.2   0.3 mile

0   0.1   0.2   0.3 kilometer

1 OLD TOWN aND CHINaTOWN: SKID row No More

BOUNDARIES: **NW Broadway, Willamette River, W. Burnside St.**
DISTANCE: **2 miles**
DIFFICULTY: **Easy**
PARKING: **Metered street parking**
PUBLIC TRANSIT: **MAX Green and Yellow Lines (Union Station), Red and Blue Lines (Old Town/Chinatown Station)**

This is the historic core of Portland, once upon a time a rough-and-tumble waterfront where sailors and loggers went carousing in the muddy streets. (Some claim it's the source of the term "Skid Row," although Seattle also claims that dubious honor—regardless, the expression refers to the path along which cut logs were ushered toward the river to be shipped.) In those days, before the harbor wall was built to help contain the waters of the Willamette River, this area flooded regularly several times a season. (This was also before an efficient sewer system had been implemented, so you can imagine.) Old Town is also home to the legendary Shanghai tunnels, where—rumor has it, though historians dispute it—drunken sailors would be dropped into tunnels below certain downtown bars, then dragged aboard ships and taken on as indentured workers. (Whether this really happened here or not, it's a good story, and you can still tour the Shanghai tunnels below town today.)

Like many urban cores, Old Town suffered from a few decades of neglect and was considered a pretty sketchy area until a few years ago, when the city's focused attention helped revitalize the neighborhood. Which isn't to say there are no longer any gritty elements, but these days, Old Town and Chinatown tend to be lively at night, with entertainment options including several good bars and clubs, art galleries, top-notch restaurants, and the Lan Su Chinese Garden, a major draw for visitors.

Part of Old Town's appeal is its historic architecture, particularly its character-rich brick and cast-iron buildings—in fact, Portland has one of the biggest collections of historic cast-iron architecture in the country. Preservation efforts have helped to keep a lot of the city's historical charm intact.

● Start at Union Station; its huge clock tower and glowing GO BY TRAIN sign make it a great landmark. It was built in 1896, not quite as commissioned by writer-turned-railway owner Henry Villard—who went bust before his plans for the station could be completed. A somewhat-more-modest version of Villard's idea was eventually built, and the interior was later remodeled by Pietro Belluschi. It's now owned and maintained by the Portland Development Commission. Attached to the station is a fittingly old-school restaurant–piano bar, Wilf's, with wingback red-velvet chairs, brick walls, chandeliers, and live jazz on the weekends.

● From Union Station, walk south along NW 6th Ave. Turn left at NW Everett and walk three blocks. At NW 3rd and Everett is Lan Su Chinese Garden. The idea of the garden was initially sparked when Portland established a sister-city relationship with Suzhou, China; gradually, momentum grew, funds were raised, and plans were made. The garden opened in September 2000, adding an important degree of solidity to the hopeful notion that Old Town was really on its way up. The garden is a tranquil and restorative place, especially remarkable considering its location, and it has that magical ability to seem much larger on the inside than it looks from the outside. There's also an adjoining tea shop where you can sample a wide range of traditional teas and light snacks.

● From Everett, turn right onto NW 2nd Ave., then right again on NW Davis. At NW 6th Ave. turn left; halfway down this block, on your right (at 125 NW 6th Ave.), was once Satyricon, the longest-running punk club on the West Coast, something like the Portland equivalent of CBGB (and similarly nonexistent today). It's hard to overestimate the importance of the club to Portland's live-music scene, and equally tough to imagine a venue today where you could see so many awesome bands in such a small space—Nirvana opened for Mudhoney here in 1989, to give just one example. The capacity was about 200 people.

Satyricon closed for good in 2010 (after having closed temporarily in 2003, turned into a soulless club called Icon, closed briefly again, then revived as an all-ages nightclub), and the building was torn down, an event that, apart from being very sad, must have smelled terrible. (Satyricon's men's room, for years, featured a communal "trough"—enough said?)

- On NW Couch St. turn left, and you'll reach Ground Kontrol, a playground for Portland-style grown-ups, a.k.a. permanent adolescents. It has all the arcade games you either remember from your youth or wish you'd had when you were a kid. The pinball collection alone is awesome. And they're all still cheap to play. There is also beer, and the space occasionally serves as a live-music venue.

- Around the corner to the left, the rest of this block is full of similarly fun enterprises, including an imported-toy store and gallery, a coffee shop–art gallery–music venue called Backspace, and an intimate music lounge. Explore at your leisure.

- At NW 5th Ave. turn right, then turn left on W. Burnside St. for a block. At Burnside and NW 4th Ave. is the 38-foot-tall Chinatown Gate, installed in 1986; turn left on 4th to pass through it. As you do, take a look across 4th Ave.; at the time of this writing, the corner block was occupied (temporarily, it seems) by a very orderly homeless camp, walled in on one side by a screen of artfully painted wooden doors along Burnside St. The camp was set up by a nonprofit organization called Right 2 Dream Too (a sign out front explains all this), which is renting the space from the landowner. It's unclear, however, what will become of the camp if the owner succeeds in selling the land or finding a tenant.

- At NW 4th Ave. and Couch St. is a good comic-book shop, Floating World, and just beyond that is the oddball 24 Hour Church of Elvis, which you really just have to experience to understand—but it's worth the tiny detour, trust us: it's a very Portland thing. Kitty-corner from Floating World is a beloved relic from a few years back, the enormous neon sign for the long-departed Chinese restaurant Hung Far Low. (It's okay if you can't keep a straight face.) Dedicated barflies adored Hung Far Low for the minuscule corner bar, dark as night, with its tiny, cheap, and powerful drinks, impassive bartenders, glowing Buddha statue, and perilously long, narrow staircase that led up from the street. When it closed (and moved to SE 82nd Ave., along with many of the businesses that once made up historic Chinatown), a touchingly sincere effort was made to preserve and keep displaying the Hung Far Low sign. It worked. (Below the sign now is a fantastic pan-Asian restaurant called Ping, worth a stop if you're at all hungry; it's co-owned by Andy Ricker, the chef behind Pok Pok.)

- Having turned right on Couch, turn right again on NW 3rd Ave., then left on W. Burnside, left again on NW 2nd Ave., and then right to get back to NW Couch. These blocks contain some of the grittier street life in the area, as well as some of the more memorable old buildings.

- Follow Couch to NW Naito Pkwy., and turn right. From here you have an interesting view of the White Stag sign, a beloved local landmark and yet another beneficiary of the Old Town preservationist spirit. (It's been changed several times to suit whichever business was using it to advertise, but the sign has now essentially been adopted by Old Town and should be safe. The large warehouse building beneath it is an example of the kind of restoration going on in this neighborhood.)

- Turn right at SW Ankeny St., where you'll see the Skidmore Fountain and Ankeny Arcade. The fountain is from 1888 and was intended for "horses, men, and dogs," but . . . drink at your own risk. This area is part of the grounds of Portland's Saturday Market, which we'll cover in Walk 10: Hawthorne Bridge to Steel Bridge.

- Continue straight ahead on SW Ankeny St. and you'll come to an alleyway shared by several bars in the block. Here again, drink at your own risk—but this is a fun and lively warm-weather hangout, and the surrounding bars are all worth investigating if it's too cold for sitting outdoors. At the corner of Ankeny and SW 3rd Ave. is the tourist favorite Voodoo Doughnut, which will most likely have a huge line outside. Go ahead—we'll be in the alley.

POINTS OF INTEREST (START TO FINISH)

Lan Su Chinese Garden portlandchinesegarden.org, 239 NW Everett St., 503-228-8131

Ground Kontrol groundkontrol.com, 511 NW Couch St., 503-796-9364

Backspace backspace.bz, 115 NW 5th Ave., 503-248-2900

Floating World Comics floatingworldcomics.com, 400 NW Couch St., 503-241-0227

24 Hour Church of Elvis 24hourchurchofelvis.com, 408 NW Couch St.

Ping pingpdx.com, 102 NW 4th Ave., 503-229-7464

Voodoo Doughnut voodoodoughnut.com, 22 SW 3rd Ave., 503-241-4704

route summary

1. Start at Union Station.
2. Walk south along NW 6th Ave.
3. Turn left on NW Everett.
4. Turn right on NW 2nd Ave.
5. Turn right on NW Davis St.
6. Turn left on NW 6th Ave.
7. Turn left on NW Couch St.
8. Turn right on NW 5th Ave.
9. Turn left on W. Burnside.
10. Turn left on NW 4th Ave.
11. Turn right on NW Couch.
12. Turn right on NW 3rd Ave.
13. Turn left on W. Burnside.
14. Turn left on NW 2nd Ave.
15. Turn right on NW Couch.
16. Turn right on NW Naito Pkwy.
17. Turn right on SW Ankeny St.

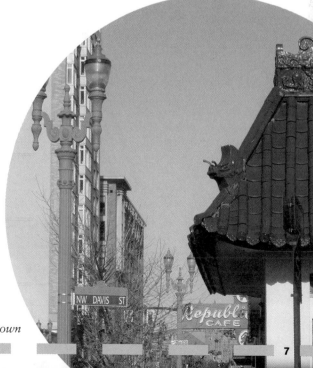

A peek into historic Old Town and Chinatown

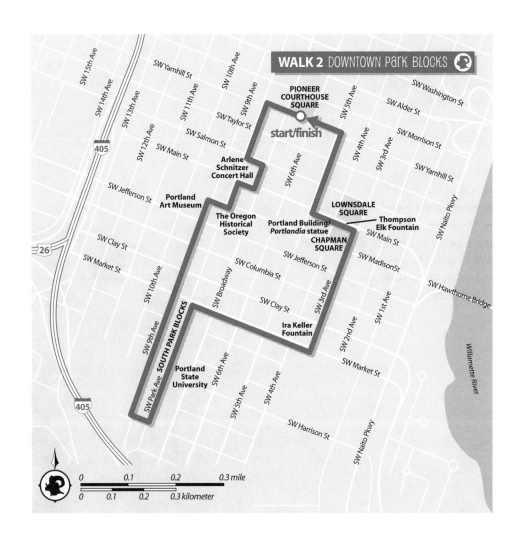

SW 15th Ave
SW 14th Ave
SW 13th Ave
SW 12th Ave
SW 11th Ave
SW 10th Ave
SW 9th Ave
SW 5th Ave
SW 4th Ave
SW 3rd Ave

SW Yamhill St
SW Washington St
SW Alder St
SW Morrison St
SW Taylor St
SW Salmon St
SW Main St
SW Jefferson St

**PIONEER
COURTHOUSE
SQUARE**

start/finish

SW Yamhill St

**Arlene
Schnitzer
Concert Hall**

SW 6th Ave

**Portland
Art Museum**

**LOWNSDALE
SQUARE**

**The Oregon
Historical
Society**

**Portland Building/
Portlandia statue**

**Thompson
Elk Fountain**

**CHAPMAN
SQUARE**

SW Main St

SW Clay St

SW Market St

SW Jefferson St

SW Columbia St

SW Madison St

SW Hawthorne Bridge

SW Broadway

SW Clay St

SW 3rd Ave

SW 2nd Ave

SW 1st Ave

SW Naito Pkwy

**Ira Keller
Fountain**

SOUTH PARK BLOCKS

SW 10th Ave

SW 9th Ave

SW Park Ave

SW 6th Ave

SW 5th Ave

SW 4th Ave

SW Market St

**Portland
State
University**

SW Harrison St

SW Naito Pkwy

Willamette River

405

26

405

0   0.1   0.2   0.3 mile
0   0.1   0.2   0.3 kilometer

2 DOWNTOWN PARK BLOCKS: MUSEUM ROW

BOUNDARIES: **SW Morrison St., SW 10th Ave., SW College St., SW 3rd Ave.**
DISTANCE: **2 miles**
DIFFICULTY: **Easy**
PARKING: **Metered street parking**
PUBLIC TRANSIT: **Nearly any TriMet Bus or MAX Light Rail line headed toward downtown**

The area generally considered Downtown Portland encompasses a pretty vast stretch of territory, but for this walk we'll stick primarily to the South Park Blocks and surrounding area—basically the city's museum district. Not only is this where you'll find the art museum and history center, it's also pleasantly removed from the bustling commercial parts of downtown. Most of the route goes along an inviting stretch of wide, traffic-free, tree-lined walkway leading toward the Portland State University campus. Before we get there, though, we'll explore the city's "living room," essentially the heart of downtown, or at least its people-watching capital: Pioneer Courthouse Square, a wide public gathering space often filled with downtown workers scarfing lunches bought from nearby food carts. It acts as an open-air event space, too, hosting concerts in summer, a farmers' market each week, annual seasonal beer fests, ethnic food and culture fairs, protests and demonstrations, book sales, and, around December, the city's enormous holiday tree.

● **Start the walk at Pioneer Courthouse Square. Horrifyingly, the square was almost turned into an 11-story parking garage instead; that's what the owners of next-door department store Meier & Frank wanted to do with the space in the 1960s, but luckily the city refused to allow it. In fact, the threat of losing an opportunity for a shared public space downtown led Portland's leaders to start developing an actual city plan, and the creation of the public square was set into motion. It opened on April 6, 1984. Today it's the site of all kinds of civic activity, everything from farmers' markets and food festivals to Occupy Wall Street protest rallies to, recently, a jam-packed Girl Talk concert. Its curved steps make a great place to sit and people-watch; the street theater here is tops.**

Among the square's many features is also one of Portland's most photographed landmarks, *Allow Me*, J. Seward Johnson's bronze statue of a man holding out his

umbrella. Under the water fountain below Starbucks—Portland's first, opened in 1989—you'll find the Travel Portland Visitor Information Center. The arched wrought-iron gate at the opposite end of the square was originally part of the Hotel Portland (see Back Story on page 12). Beyond the gate and across the street is the historic Pioneer Courthouse, which opened in 1875 and serves the U.S. Courts' 9th Circuit.

● Take SW Yamhill St. one block to SW Park Ave. and turn left. At SW Salmon St. turn left again, then turn right onto SW Broadway. This block is dominated by the Arlene Schnitzer Concert Hall and its epic neon PORTLAND sign, which used to say PARAMOUNT. If you hesitate to walk underneath it, your fears are not unfounded: in the mid-1980s, the PARAMOUNT sign fell to the street during a disassembly and was replaced with the current PORTLAND sign). "The Schnitz," as it's called, is the home of the Oregon Symphony and several other performing-arts groups. Originally a vaudeville hall, then a movie house (the Paramount), then a concert venue, it's now a great place to see just about any performance. The ornate Italian Rococo Revival interior and romantic lighting make even the most mundane lecture seem fancy.

● Turn right up SW Main St. and then left on Park Ave. to reach The Oregon Historical Society. In addition to a stellar Oregon history–themed bookshop and an extensive archive of photos, maps, and documents, the OHS is also a museum with exhibits about various periods from the state's history. Objects and artifacts on display include Oregon's first car, the Benson auto, cobbled together in a garage in 1904; meeting minutes from the earliest days of the Emanuel Hospital board, written in Swedish; and a massive guestbook from the Lewis and Clark Centennial Expo in 1905 (so huge it gets wheeled around in its own custom-made transporter box). There's also a gallery of Northwest art, an exploration of the state's geology, and temporary exhibits.

● Across the South Park Blocks from the OHS is the Portland Art Museum. PAM was founded in 1892; by 1913 it had gained enough traction to be one of the stops on the tour of the New York Armory Show, which rocked the art world of the time. The museum complex includes a number of buildings and galleries, as well as the Northwest Film Center. Don't neglect to stop by the highly regarded Vivian and Gordon Gilkey Center for Graphic Arts; its permanent collection includes 30 prints donated by Robert Rauschenberg in 1976. (Rauschenberg's son, Christopher, is a photographer who lives in the area and is an active figure in the arts community, having cofounded two Portland galleries himself.) The Northwest Film Center schedule is also worth checking; its programs often include hard-to-find films, sometimes with director Q&As afterward, and the theater is pristine. The film center runs the hugely popular annual Portland International Film Festival each winter.

- After you've left the museum, take the opportunity to stroll all the way to the end of the South Park Blocks. When the pedestrian walkway peters out toward the far side of the Portland State campus, make two lefts to cross to the other side of the South Park Blocks and come back toward town, staying on SW Park Ave. At SW Market St., turn right, then turn left at SW 3rd Ave. to swing by the Ira Keller Fountain, the centerpiece of Keller Fountain Park. It's a great place to hang out on a hot day; the intersecting planes of the waterfall are Tetris-level entrancing, and it's tucked away just enough off the main drag to feel like an escape from downtown traffic.

- Follow SW 3rd Ave. to Main St. and turn left to walk between Lownsdale Square and Chapman Square; this was the nexus of Portland's Occupy Wall Street movement. Folks were camped out here for weeks during the OWS protests of summer 2012, but eventually city authorities forced them to leave.

Also on SW Main St., between 3rd and 4th Aves., is the Thompson Elk Fountain, which as anyone can see is facing the wrong direction, with its back to the oncoming cars, bikes, and buses. It has stood here since 1900, when, presumably, traffic was a little less streamlined.

Ahead of you on the left side of Main St.—and possibly the object of the Thompson Elk's disapproving gaze—is the much-maligned Portland Building. It holds city offices and meeting rooms, and it looks like a really big Christmas present nobody wants to find under the tree. (This opinion isn't terribly controversial; the Portland Building served as the lead example in a 2009 *Travel + Leisure* magazine article titled "World's Ugliest Buildings," if that tells you anything.) Designed by Michael Graves and opened in 1982, it is usually considered the first major postmodern building in the country. Perched over the front entrance is the (much more attractive, if also a bit intimidating) bronze statue *Portlandia,* by Raymond Kaskey. His design was selected by a committee, which included Graves, to complement the building's design. After the Statue of Liberty, *Portlandia* is the largest hammered-copper statue in the United States. If she

Back Story: Hotel Portland

Though it would eventually become known as the most fabulous building ever to grace the city, the Hotel Portland had a troubled start. It was dreamed up in 1882 by Henry Villard, the railroad boss who built Union Station and is generally credited with getting a transcontinental rail line to Portland. But Villard went broke and high-tailed it back to his native Germany before the hotel could be finished. It took a couple of years and about 150 other investors, including William S. Ladd, Henry Failing, George Markle, and Henry Corbett, to wrap up construction on the project. The total cost was over $1 million.

The Hotel Portland (or Portland Hotel, depending on which antique postcard you're looking at) finally opened in 1890 and was by all accounts very posh, if a bit on the sturdy-and-stodgy side. It quickly became the cultural centerpiece of the city, with its elegant dining rooms and ballrooms. Eleven U.S. presidents stayed there.

But its glory had begun to fade by the 1940s, when Meier & Frank bought the building; it was torn down in 1951 for parking space, which was eventually replaced by Pioneer Courthouse Square. The original wrought-iron gate from the hotel now stands at one end of the square.

stood up from her perch, she'd be the 50-Foot Woman. (Even crouched, she's 36 feet tall.) *Portlandia* traveled to her current location by barge along the Willamette River and was installed in 1985. (A few years later, local developer Joseph Weston offered to pay with his own money to have the statue moved to Waterfront Park, where people could see it without, as he put it, worrying about being hit by a bus, but the city declined his offer.)

● Take SW Main St. to SW 5th Ave. and turn right. Follow 5th Ave. to SW Yamhill St. and turn left to return to Pioneer Courthouse Square.

POINTS OF INTEREST (START TO FINISH)

Travel Portland Visitor Information Center travelportland.com, 701 SW 6th Ave., 503-275-8355

Arlene Schnitzer Concert Hall pcpa.com/schnitzer, 1037 SW Broadway, 503-248-4335

The Oregon Historical Society ohs.org, 1200 SW Park Ave., 503-222-1741

Portland Art Museum pam.org, 1219 SW Park Ave., 503-226-2811

Portland Building 1120 SW 5th Ave.

ROUTE SUMMARY

1. Start at Pioneer Courthouse Square.
2. From SW Yamhill St., turn left onto SW Park Ave.
3. Turn left at SW Salmon St.
4. Turn right on SW Broadway.
5. Turn right on SW Main St.
6. Turn left on SW Park Ave.
7. Cross South Park Blocks to the Portland Art Museum.
8. Walk to the end of the South Park Blocks, making two lefts to cross the blocks and then head back toward town on SW Park Ave.
9. Turn right at SW Market St.
10. Turn left at SW 3rd Ave.
11. Turn left at SW Main St.
12. Turn right at SW 5th Ave.
13. Turn left at SW Yamhill St.

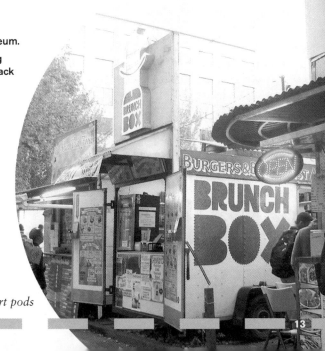

One of Portland's many food-cart pods

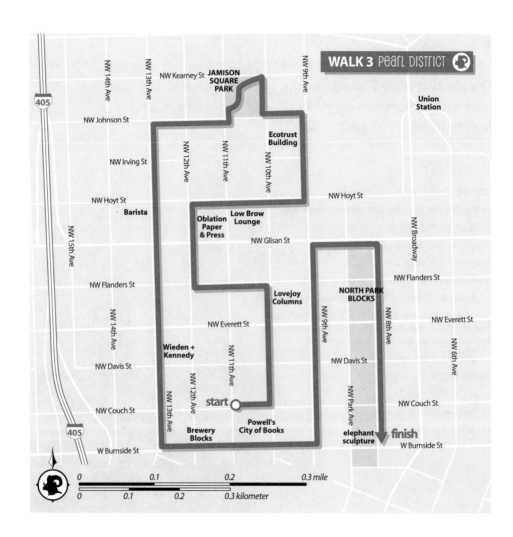

NW 14th Ave

NW 13th Ave

NW Kearney St

JAMISON SQUARE PARK

NW 9th Ave

Union Station

NW Johnson St

Ecotrust Building

NW Irving St

NW 12th Ave

NW 11th Ave

NW 10th Ave

NW Hoyt St

Barista

NW 15th Ave

Oblation Paper & Press

Low Brow Lounge

NW Hoyt St

NW Broadway

NW Glisan St

NW Flanders St

Lovejoy Columns

NORTH PARK BLOCKS

NW Flanders St

NW 14th Ave

NW Everett St

NW 9th Ave

NW 8th Ave

NW Everett St

NW 6th Ave

Wieden + Kennedy

NW 11th Ave

NW Davis St

NW Davis St

NW Park Ave

NW Couch St

NW 12th Ave

start

NW Couch St

NW 13th Ave

Powell's City of Books

elephant sculpture

finish

Brewery Blocks

W Burnside St

W Burnside St

0   0.1   0.2   0.3 mile

0   0.1   0.2   0.3 kilometer

3 Pearl District: Urban Art Project

BOUNDARIES: **NW Lovejoy St., NW Couch St., NW 15th Ave., NW Broadway**
DISTANCE: **2 miles**
DIFFICULTY: **Easy**
PARKING: **On street**
PUBLIC TRANSIT: **TriMet Bus 20 (W. Burnside and NW Park Ave.) or Portland Streetcar (NW 11th Ave. and Couch St., NW 11th Ave. and Glisan St.)**

The Pearl District hasn't always been the urban-designer's dream zone it is today. Until about 15 years or so ago, it wasn't really known as anything at all—sort of a blank, vaguely forbidding area between downtown and NW 23rd Avenue, full of empty warehouses and vacant lots. (At a recent live show with his band the Afghan Whigs in Portland recently, musician Greg Dulli told the crowd, "I've been coming to Portland since the '80s. There was *not* a Whole Foods in the Pearl in the '80s.") Gradually, a small vanguard of artists, drawn as ever by the cheap rent in out-of-the-way loft spaces, started moving in. Around the same time (roughly, the late 1980s and early 1990s), the Portland Development Commission noticed the area—the smart money always follows the artists. By 2000 the Pearl District had officially become a "project." In October 2001 the City Council voted to adopt the "Pearl District Development Plan: A Future Vision for a Neighborhood in Transition."

And boy, did that ever work. These days the Pearl is the kind of neighborhood you have to get dressed up for. Those empty warehouses are now sleekly renovated lofts and condos, and the streets are lined with upscale galleries, home-decor shops, and high-end restaurants. The Portland Streetcar carries people in from downtown (although it's often faster just to walk). Once a month the district becomes a huge street party during the First Thursday Art Walk, when galleries open their doors to premiere new exhibits. (Some people do actually go to look at the art, though many are there to check each other out—and for the free wine.) Some locals love to hate the Pearl—it's too moneyed and too polished to be interesting, and rent is way beyond a struggling artist's budget—but certainly from an urban-planning perspective, the transformation is remarkable.

● Start the walk from NW 11th Ave. and Couch St., where there's a Portland Streetcar stop. Walk east down Couch for a block, noting the rear entrance of Powell's Books on your right—don't worry, we'll come back to Powell's—then turn left on NW 10th Ave.

● In a courtyard between NW Everett and Flanders Sts., on your right, you'll find the installation of the two remaining Lovejoy Columns. These columns, which held up the ramp from NW Lovejoy St. onto the Broadway Bridge before it was demolished, were rescued by a hard-fought civic battle. Artist Tom Stefopoulos, who was a watchman at one of the nearby train yards in the 1940s, had embellished the columns during slow nights at work, and his paintings had become a favorite local landmark. When developers decided to tear down the Lovejoy Ramp in the late 1990s to make room for more of the Pearl, there was huge debate over what to do about the columns. For a while they lay in an empty lot, wrapped in tarps, awaiting their fate. Finally, developer John Carroll offered to install the two main columns in the plaza outside his Elizabeth Tower apartment building, and there they stand today. Whatever you make of the artwork, the inspired effort that went into preserving it—not to mention the awesome spectacle of those massive columns ripped free, their rebar guts exposed to the air—is damned impressive.

● From NW 10th Ave., turn left on NW Flanders St., then right on NW 12th Ave. If, like us, you're a sucker for fancy paper shops, stop in at Oblation Papers & Press, on the right-hand side of the street. (Of course, there are galleries and shops throughout this area; let your curiosity guide you.)

● At NW Hoyt St., turn right. At Hoyt and NW 10th Ave. you'll find one of the few entirely unpretentious bars (maybe the only one?) in the Pearl—the Low Brow Lounge. It has somehow held out against the forces of commerce and fashion, sticking to its supercheap guns. It's impenetrably dark when you first walk in, but you'll adjust. Once you do, look around for the tiny "makeout booth" in the far corner. Plus: black lights!

● Continue along NW Hoyt St. and, at NW 9th Ave., turn left to pass behind the Ecotrust Building (corner of 9th and NW Johnson St.). Turn left on NW Johnson St. The Ecotrust Building, formally known as the Jean Vollum Natural Capital Center, is a hundred-year-old warehouse that was among the first in the area to be transformed into something new. When its remodel was finished in 2001, the

U.S. Green Building Center gave it a LEED Gold rating, the first ever for a restoration of a historic building. Its design, which even those indifferent to architecture can appreciate, preserves the look and texture of the original (including some of the walls around the parking area, rough edges and all) and includes an ecoroof and a set of solar panels that provide 10% of the building's energy supply. In short, it's a pretty cool building, and is one of the reasons people got so excited about what was going on in the Pearl District when the wave of warehouse renovations began. (There's also a really good pizza joint inside: Hotlips, which uses all-local organic ingredients.)

● From NW Johnson St., take a right on NW 10th Ave., then a left on NW Kearney St., to reach Jamison Square Park. When the park first appeared it was a little, um, stark: essentially a featureless concrete disc with a fountain in the middle. But it quickly grew into itself and now feels more like an urban oasis, with shade trees and seating areas around the fountain. It's wildly popular, especially with the parents of little kids, so it can get hectic on weekends and summer afternoons. But it definitely helps make the neighborhood seem like a place where people actually live, rather than just a theoretical exercise in how one might live. (The park is named after William Jamison, a universally adored Portland art gallery owner who died in 1995.)

● Cross the square diagonally, emerging at NW 11th Ave. and NW Johnson St., and take a right onto Johnson. At NW 13th Ave. turn left. This strip has a number of very highly rated restaurants, if you're feeling peckish. And for the coffee addicts, between NW Hoyt and Glisan is Barista, where you can get an impeccably pulled espresso shot and great advice on choosing a bag of beans to take home with you.

● Between Everett and Davis on NW 13th Ave. is the Portland headquarters of the Wieden + Kennedy ad agency, which runs prominent campaigns for Nike and Old Spice, among others. The building is yet another astounding renovation of an old warehouse (from 1908). Even the front doors are intimidating.

● From NW 13th, turn left on W. Burnside St. This area was once home to the Henry Weinhard Brewery blocks. (Note the slick, newish Henry's 12th Street Tavern, a block down.) Weinhard ran a beer empire from here for decades. He made so much beer and distributed it so widely that at one point he supposedly offered to just go ahead and pump the lager directly into Skidmore Fountain, so everybody could have some.

The brewery produced 100,000 barrels of beer a year in 1890. And, remarkably, it survived Prohibition, temporarily adapting to the times with "near beer." But nothing lasts forever: in 1979, what was by then Blitz-Weinhard was sold to Pabst, and Pabst sold it to Stroh's in 1996. Three years later Stroh's sold the brand to Miller Brewing Co., and that was the end of Weinhard's brewing in the brewery blocks. (Henry Weinhard's beer is still made today, but in the Olympia Brewery in Tumwater, Washington.)

● Follow W. Burnside St. a few more blocks to NW 10th Ave. and the main entrance of Powell's City of Books. As you'll know from having just seen the back side of it, the place is massive—a whole city block and multiple levels of new, used, and rare books and magazines. Go on in and plan to stay awhile. (Powell's also has regular author readings—check its website for a schedule.)

● After you leave Powell's, continue along W. Burnside St. and turn left on NW 9th Ave. This stretch includes another series of art galleries to explore. At NW Glisan St., turn right, then right again on NW 8th Ave. to walk along the North Park Blocks. Between NW Davis and Couch Sts. is another building containing several galleries and the Museum of Contemporary Craft. Affiliated with the Pacific Northwest College of Art, it has both permanent and changing exhibitions.

● At the far end of the North Park Blocks, between NW Couch and W. Burnside Sts., is a 12-foot bronze sculpture of an elephant carrying a smaller elephant on its back. This is a gift from a Chinese businessman whose bronze foundry is licensed to reproduce Chinese antiquities. The elephant is modeled after a much-smaller Shang dynasty wine pitcher. (No wine inside this one, though, alas.)

● From here, return to W. Burnside St., where you can catch a bus or walk a few blocks farther to downtown.

Back story: esther Lovejoy

An early example of a tough Portland woman, Esther Lovejoy got a medical degree at the University of Oregon in 1894, graduating with honors. She married and had a son with a fellow med-school student, but both the son and the husband had died by 1911. Esther went on to marry a local businessman, George Lovejoy, but they were divorced in 1920. Before all of that, though, Portland's mayor appointed Esther to the city board of health. Two years later she became city health officer, the first woman to have such a major civic role in any large US city. She made it a priority to crack down on poor hygiene, particularly in schools and in terms of the city's garbage-collection practices, and she emphasized good-quality food and milk. She was also a fierce advocate for women's right to control their own lives; among other things, this included advocating for the right to vote. Oregon women achieved suffrage in 1912, but Esther didn't stop there; she continued to organize and fight for the right to vote on a national level. She wrote and published several books about the history of women in medicine. She also worked for public health improvements in poor and neglected areas overseas. She served as director of the international relief organization American Women's Hospitals from 1919 until she died in 1967.

POINTS OF INTEREST (START TO FINISH)

Oblation Papers & Press oblationpapers.com, 516 NW 12th Ave., 503-223-1093

Low Brow Lounge 1036 NW Hoyt St., 503-226-0200

Ecotrust Building 721 NW 9th Ave.

Hotlips hotlipspizza.com, NW 10th Ave. and Irving St., 503-595-2342

Barista baristapdx.com, 539 NW 13th Ave.

Wieden + Kennedy wk.com, 224 NW 13th Ave., 503-937-7000

Powell's City of Books powells.com, 1005 W. Burnside St., 503-228-4651

Museum of Contemporary Craft museumofcontemporarycraft.org, 724 NW Davis St., 503-223-2654

route summary

1. Start at the corner of NW 11th Ave. and Couch St.; walk east on Couch.
2. Turn left on NW 10th Ave.
3. Turn left on NW Flanders St.
4. Turn right on NW 12th Ave.
5. Turn right on NW Hoyt St.
6. Turn left on NW 9th Ave.
7. Turn left on NW Johnson St.
8. Turn right on NW 10th Ave.
9. Turn left on NW Kearney St.
10. Walk diagonally across Jamison Square Park.
11. Turn right on NW Johnson St.
12. Turn left on NW 13th Ave.
13. Turn left on W. Burnside St.
14. Turn left on NW 9th Ave.
15. Turn right on NW Glisan St.
16. Turn right on NW 8th Ave.
16. Take NW 8th Ave. to W. Burnside St.

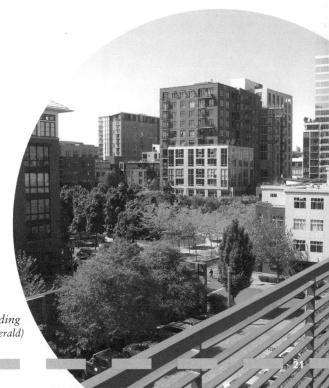

View of Pearl District from the Ecotrust Building
(Photo courtesy of Paul Gerald)

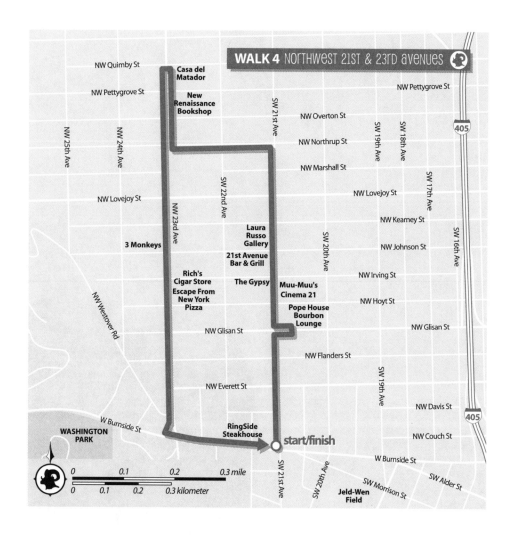

NW Quimby St

NW Pettygrove St

NW Pettygrove St

Casa del Matador

New Renaissance Bookshop

SW 21st Ave

NW Overton St

NW Northrup St

NW Marshall St

SW 19th Ave

SW 18th Ave

405

NW 25th Ave

NW 24th Ave

NW Lovejoy St

NW Lovejoy St

SW 17th Ave

NW 23rd Ave

SW 22nd Ave

NW Kearney St

SW 16th Ave

3 Monkeys

Laura Russo Gallery

21st Avenue Bar & Grill

NW Johnson St

SW 20th Ave

NW Irving St

Rich's Cigar Store

Escape From New York Pizza

The Gypsy

Muu-Muu's Cinema 21

Pope House Bourbon Lounge

NW Hoyt St

NW Westover Rd

NW Glisan St

NW Glisan St

NW Flanders St

NW Everett St

SW 19th Ave

NW Davis St

405

WASHINGTON PARK

W Burnside St

RingSide Steakhouse

start/finish

NW Couch St

W Burnside St

SW Alder St

0   0.1   0.2   0.3 mile

0   0.1   0.2   0.3 kilometer

SW 21st Ave

SW 20th Ave

SW Morrison St

Jeld-Wen Field

4 Northwest 21st and 23rd avenues: Faded Glamour

BOUNDARIES: **W. Burnside St., NW Raleigh St., NW 20th Ave., NW 24th Ave.**
DISTANCE: **2 miles**
DIFFICULTY: **Easy**
PARKING: **Free street parking (with time limits)**
PUBLIC TRANSIT: **TriMet Bus 20 (W. Burnside St. and NW King Ave.)**

Northwest (the general term for 21st and 23rd Avenues and the surrounding blocks) has seen easier times. Once considered the fanciest and most desirable part of Portland, it's now frequently mocked (NW 23rd has long sported the obvious nickname "Trendy-third") by people who live on the other side of the river; the glam boutiques and upscale restaurants that defined it went either out of style or out of business as unemployment grew and disposable income shrank. For years this was the undebated first stop for any serious eating, drinking, or shopping to be done in Portland, but as the city has matured and other neighborhoods have taken over as talked-up destinations, Northwest has seemed to fade a little. In urban-planning magazine articles it's outshined by the neighboring Pearl District, and in youth-approved cool it loses out to Old Town, Alberta, and much of Southeast. Still, there's a lingering Euro-style beauty to the tree-lined streets and vintage buildings, and there are plenty of other reasons to seek out this area: one of the greatest art-house cinemas in the country, for one thing, not to mention a killer gourmet-grocery market, an appropriately cranky New York–style pizza joint, and several places in which one can sip a cocktail and feel like an adult. Plus the whole thing is part of the Alphabet Historic District, which is listed on the National Register of Historic Places and boasts some lovely residential buildings.

● **Start at the corner of W. Burnside St. and NW 21st Ave., heading north along 21st. The junior of the two main streets in Northwest is also the mellower one, with, generally speaking, more laid-back hangouts and fewer upscale shops.**

● **If you duck down NW Glisan St., to the right and two doors down, you'll come to the very pretty Pope House Bourbon Lounge, a bar inside a Victorian mansion that once housed the late, lamented Brazen Bean. (The Bean was a cocktail lounge of the sort that practically guaranteed your date would go well—it was one of the first cool, stylish places to get masterfully crafted grown-up cocktails in Portland.) The**

Pope House has a gorgeous outdoor garden for fair-weather seating, plus many shelves of whiskey, hardwood floors, and a rifle behind the bar inside.

- Go back up Glisan to NW 21st Ave. and take a right. Just past NW Hoyt St. you'll come to Cinema 21, one of the best movie theaters left standing (in Portland or anywhere). It's a single-screen theater from the 1960s that now shows top-notch art-house films, and whatever it has booked is always worth checking out (with the possible exception of *The Room,* the inexplicably popular *Rocky Horror*–like movie that screens here once a month). Cinema 21 also frequently holds well-chosen revivals, recently including a night of Bogart classics, several days of second-tier but still great film-noir titles, and a week or so of Hitchcock movies—in 35 mm, of course. And it's the headquarters for a number of local and regional film festivals. Seats are supercomfy, and beer and wine are now available.

- Continuing along NW 21st Ave., you'll find an ever-shifting lineup of restaurants and bars, some of which have been around forever (The Gypsy; the 21st Avenue Bar & Grill, with the unlikeliest of secret gardens on its lovely back patio) and many that will have vanished and reappeared in another incarnation by the time this book hits shelves. One of the better choices is Muu-Muu's, next door to Cinema 21, for good food and drinks in a cozy, only slightly kitschy atmosphere.

- Just past NW Johnson St., on the left, is the Laura Russo Gallery. Russo died in 2010, but the gallery, established in 1986, continues to be an important fixture in the Portland art scene (after Russo died, her longtime assistant took over running the gallery and has kept it pretty much the same). Russo was a major player in bringing wider attention to some of the most important artists of the Pacific Northwest, and the gallery helped establish many of the region's big names, including Henk Pander, Lucinda Parker, Tom Cramer, and Mary Josephson. Stop in for an efficient lesson in the art of the region, past and present.

- At NW Northrup St., turn left, then take a right onto NW 23rd Ave. Just past NW Overton St. you'll see the huge, vividly pastel confection that is the New Renaissance Bookshop, a new-age bookstore occupying three storefronts. Pick up a meditation calendar or some wind chimes, or maybe have your aura decontaminated. Seriously, just *try* to be grouchy in here—it can't be done.

- A little farther down the street, at NW Quimby St., is a more appropriate receptacle for scorn: the Casa del Matador, almost universally referred to as "the cougar bar" in reference to its regular crowd, which consists largely of fabulous-looking, shimmery-topped women of a certain age who may or may not be on the prowl. In short, it's the sort of thing you'll like if you like that sort of thing. If not, this is a good place to cross Quimby St. and turn left to head south along NW 23rd Ave., back the way you came.

- There are tons of interesting and horrible shops along NW 23rd, but one of the most longstanding and worth poking around in is 3 Monkeys, between NW Kearney and Johnson Sts. It sells funky clothes, jewelry, gifts, accessories, and knicknacks of all kinds. Farther along, between NW Flanders and Everett Sts., are a handful of kitchen and home-furnishings shops.

- At Irving you'll find yet another of this neighborhood's destination retailers: Rich's Cigar Store, which along with cigars has one of the better magazine selections in town, including lots of imports you can't find anywhere else (well, anywhere except Rich's other locations). There's a huge plastic horse out front. Do not touch it.

- Between NW Irving and Hoyt Sts. is the excellent Escape From New York Pizza, the first (and for some, the only) by-the-slice pizza place in Portland. Escape From New York churns out classic thin-crust pie with attitude: service is usually grumpy, there aren't many choices, they don't take credit cards, and they won't give you ranch dressing. (Why would you ask for ranch dressing?) Get a slice, fold it, walk around. Forget you ever even heard of New Renaissance Bookshop.

- At W. Burnside St., hang a left for a couple of blocks until you reach RingSide Steakhouse. Even if you're stuffed with New York pizza, it's worth stopping in here for an artfully poured cocktail at the tiny, sunken bar. The RingSide is old-school Portland: a classy but not stuffy steakhouse with flawless service and an unbelievable happy-hour menu (even on Sundays!). The place has been here since 1944 but underwent a thorough remodel in 2010, leaving all the charming touches (like a crooked fireplace) unchanged but adding kitchen space and a 10,000-square-foot wine cellar in the basement.

- The bus stop where your walk began is right across the street.

POINTS OF INTEREST (START TO FINISH)

Pope House Bourbon Lounge popehouselounge.com, 2075 NW Glisan St., 503-222-1056

Cinema 21 cinema21.com, 616 NW 21st Ave., 503-223-4515

The Gypsy cegportland.com/gypsy, 625 NW 21st Ave., 503-796-1859

21st Avenue Bar & Grill 21stbarandgrill.com, 721 NW 21st Ave., 503-222-4121

Muu-Muu's muumuus.net, 612 NW 21st Ave., 503-223-8196

Laura Russo Gallery laurarusso.com, 805 NW 21st Ave., 503-226-2754

New Renaissance Bookshop newrenbooks.com, 1338 NW 23rd Ave., 503-224-4929

Casa del Matador 1438 NW 23rd Ave., 503-228-2855

3 Monkeys 811 NW 23rd Ave., 503-222-5160

Rich's Cigar Store richscigar.com, 706 NW 23rd Ave., 503-227-6907

Escape From New York Pizza efnypizza.net, 622 NW 23rd Ave., 503-227-5423

RingSide Steakhouse ringsidesteakhouse.com, 2165 W. Burnside St., 503-223-1513

ROUTE SUMMARY

1. Start at the corner of W. Burnside St. and NW 21st Ave.

2. Walk north on NW 21st Ave.

3. Turn right at NW Glisan and walk half a block.

4. Return to NW 21st Ave. and turn right.

5. Turn left on NW Northrup St.

6. Turn right at NW 23rd Ave.

7. At NW Quimby St., turn left to cross the street and reverse course.

8. Turn left on NW 23rd Ave.

9. Turn left at W. Burnside St.

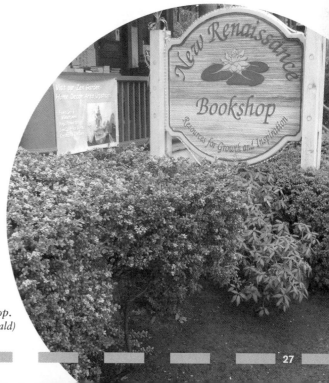

Decompress at New Renaissance Bookshop.
  (Photo courtesy of Paul Gerald)

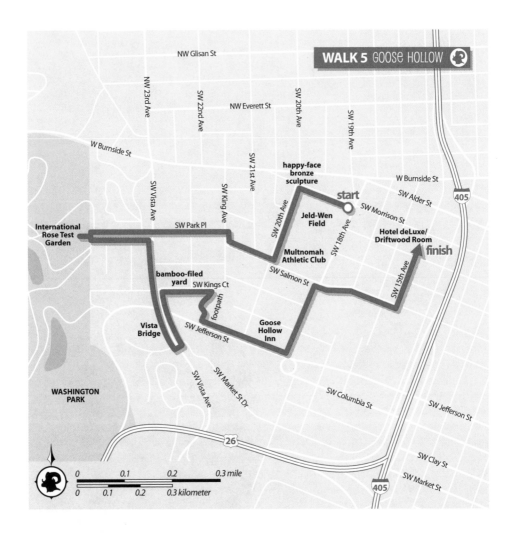

NW Glisan St

NW 23rd Ave

SW 22nd Ave

NW Everett St

SW 20th Ave

SW 19th Ave

W Burnside St

SW 21st Ave

happy-face bronze sculpture

W Burnside St

SW Alder St

405

SW Vista Ave

SW King Ave

SW 20th Ave

start

SW Morrison St

Jeld-Wen Field

SW 18th Ave

Hotel deLuxe/ Driftwood Room

International Rose Test Garden

SW Park Pl

Multnomah Athletic Club

finish

bamboo-filed yard

SW Kings Ct

SW Salmon St

SW 15th Ave

footpath

Vista Bridge

SW Jefferson St

Goose Hollow Inn

WASHINGTON PARK

SW Vista Ave

SW Market St Dr

SW Columbia St

SW Jefferson St

26

SW Clay St

405

SW Market St

0   0.1   0.2   0.3 mile

0   0.1   0.2   0.3 kilometer

5 GOOSE HOLLOW: THIS BUD'S FOR YOU

BOUNDARIES: **I-405, W. Burnside St., SW Jefferson St., Washington Park**
DISTANCE: **2 miles**
DIFFICULTY: **Moderate–strenuous (hilly in places)**
PARKING: **Free street parking**
PUBLIC TRANSIT: **TriMet Bus 15 (SW Morrison St. and 16th Ave.), MAX Red and Blue Lines (Jeld-Wen Field Station)**

Goose Hollow as an entity actually predates incorporated Portland by about six years. Daniel Lownsdale, who built the first house here, ran a tannery on the site that became Civic Stadium (now Jeld-Wen Field, home of the beloved Portland Timbers soccer team). Years later, the area was named for the flocks of geese that used to roam around here—although you'd be forgiven for thinking it's because of the cozy and well-loved Goose Hollow Inn, the pub that former mayor Bud Clark has owned here since 1967. When Clark first opened the place, the neighborhood hadn't quite established a strong sense of identity, so Clark gave his pub a historical name in hopes of reviving the Goose Hollow spirit. This apparently worked like a charm, as the name has stuck since the 1970s and the neighborhood seems to have coalesced around it.

● Start at SW Morrison St. and 18th Ave., at the corner of Jeld-Wen Field. Walk up Morrison alongside the stadium. At SW 20th Ave., turn left—but not before taking note of the remarkably disturbing happy-face bronze sculpture at the corner, one of a matched pair, presumably intended to keep the faint of heart from entering the stadium to watch a game.

● On your left as you walk up the hill, you have a chance to peer down at folks in the exclusive Multnomah Athletic Club doing their workouts. (Hey, if they didn't want anyone to look, they wouldn't have put windows there.) Turn right on SW Salmon St., then right again briefly on SW King Ave.; then make a quick left onto SW Park Pl. The houses up here are enormous and beautiful, with tons of character.

● Continue up SW Park Pl. all the way to the point at which it dead-ends in stairs leading up to a garden. If you're so inclined, you can continue along this path to reach the Washington Park International Rose Test Garden. (And, if you like, you could also link up with the Washington Park walk, page 35.) It's a pretty serious climb, but you're rewarded with an amazing view from the top. Otherwise, simply climb as many stairs as you feel like, have a look around, and head back along SW Park Pl. the way you came.

- At SW Vista Ave., turn right. This leads to the Vista Bridge, an underrated Portland viewpoint. The bridge, which stretches over busy SW Jefferson St. and the MAX Light Rail tracks heading west toward Hillsboro, is rather morbidly nicknamed the Suicide Bridge due to the number of people who've jumped from it. Even so, the view across Portland from the middle of the bridge is fantastic, especially at sunset, and the little details of the bridge's embellishments—gargoyles, lanterns, iron spires— add a nice Gothic touch.

- Cross back over the bridge and turn right on SW Kings Ct. This is a narrow one-way street, with traffic going the other way, so be alert—but don't miss the yard filled entirely with a whispering forest of bamboo plants, on your left-hand side as you start down the hill. Toward the bottom of the hill, just before Kings Ct. swerves left to become SW King Ave., a small concrete footpath leads off to the right, down a hill between two houses. Follow its zigzag pattern to the bot-tom of the hill, emerging at SW Jefferson St., and hang a left on Jefferson.

- At the corner of SW 19th Ave. and Jefferson St. is the Goose Hollow Inn, run by former mayor Bud Clark (who can frequently be seen hanging out there). It's an extremely cozy little pub, with a great wooden deck, friendly servers, hearty pizza, and a famously good Reuben sandwich.

- Where SW Jefferson St. meets SW 18th Ave., turn left. Follow SW 18th to the stoplight at SW Salmon St. and cross, turning right on Salmon.

- At SW 15th Ave., turn left. Just past SW Yamhill St. you'll come to the Hotel deLuxe, formerly the Mallory, a very nicely renovated boutique hotel whose tiny 1950s-style bar, the Driftwood Room, is a cocktail connoisseur's dream. The snappily dressed folks behind the bar work magic here—put yourself in their tender care, and you won't regret it. (Plenty of others are in on the secret, though, and the bar is really small, so it's best to come on a weeknight or right when the place opens.)

Back Story: Bud Clark, "The People's Mayor"

Bud Clark was just a folksy tavern owner when he ran for mayor against incumbent Frank Ivancie in 1984. Ivancie was a former city commissioner, a formidable and well-connected career politician who had already secured endorsements from many of the city's most powerful groups and institutions, including labor unions and *The Oregonian*. (Trivia: It was Ivancie who, as part of his 1982 "war on crime" agenda, made it illegal to give Portland police officers the middle finger.) Clark, on the other hand, was known mainly for having flashed a statue of a nude woman in the now-iconic "Expose Yourself to Art" poster. It should've been a joke of a campaign, and that's more or less how Ivancie's people decided to treat it. But against the odds, and most observers' predictions, Clark won—by a wide margin—thanks in large part to his grassroots campaigning and his folksy, man-of-the-people style.

Clark served as mayor for eight years. His accomplishments while in office include formulating the city's first-ever 12-point plan for ending homelessness; leading development of the Oregon Convention Center; introducing the city to community policing; and sponsoring the Mayor's Ball, a fund-raising live music concert that had the pleasing side effect of helping to solidify the indie music scene in Portland. Today the city's new transitional housing and community resource center for the homeless is named Bud Clark Commons in honor of the former mayor.

● The walk ends here; catch MAX Light Rail just around the corner, on either SW Yamhill or SW Morrison depending on which way you're heading. (It's also a short, easy walk from here to the 5th Ave.–6th Ave. Transit Mall downtown.)

POINTS OF INTEREST (START TO FINISH)

Jeld-Wen Field jeld-wenfield.com, SE Morrison St. and 18th Ave.

Goose Hollow Inn goosehollowinn.com, 1927 SW Jefferson St., 503-228-7010

Driftwood Room graciesdining.com/driftwood.html, 729 SW 15th Ave., 503-222-2171

route summary

1. Start at SW Morrison St. and 18th Ave.
2. Take SW Morrison to the corner of the stadium.
3. Turn left on SW 20th Ave.
4. Turn right on SW Salmon St.
5. Turn right on SW King Ave.
6. Turn left at SW Park Pl.
7. At the end of SW Park Pl., turn and retrace your steps.
8. Turn right at SW Vista Ave.
9. Cross the Vista Bridge, then retrace your steps back across.
10. Turn right on SW Kings Ct.
11. Turn right at the footpath down the hill.
12. Turn left on SW Jefferson St.
13. Turn left on SW 18th Ave.
14. Turn right on SW Salmon St.
15. Turn left on SW 15th Ave.

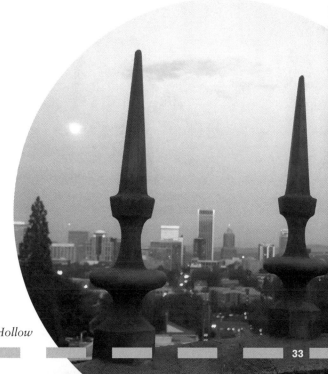

View of downtown from the Vista Bridge in Goose Hollow

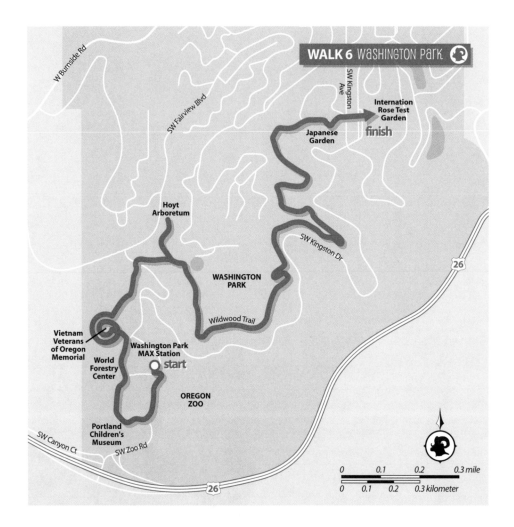

WALK 6 Washington Park

W Burnside Rd

SW Fairview Blvd

SW Kingston Ave

International
Rose Test
Garden

finish

Japanese
Garden

Hoyt
Arboretum

SW Kingston Dr

26

WASHINGTON
PARK

Wildwood Trail

Vietnam
Veterans
of Oregon
Memorial

Washington Park
MAX Station

start

World
Forestry
Center

OREGON
ZOO

Portland
Children's
Museum

SW Canyon Ct

SW Zoo Rd

26

| 0 | 0.1 | 0.2 | 0.3 mile |
| 0 | 0.1 | 0.2 | 0.3 kilometer |

6 WashiNGTON Park: LIONS, TODDLers, aNd Trees

BOUNDARIES: **W. Burnside St., SW Vista Ave., SW Sunset Hwy., SW Skyline Blvd.**
DISTANCE: **3 miles, with options to extend**
DIFFICULTY: **Easy–moderate**
PARKING: **Lots (some with a fee)**
PUBLIC TRANSIT: **MAX Red and Blue Lines (Washington Park Station), TriMet Bus 83 (SW Kingston Ave. and Japanese Garden)**

Yet another of the many things that make Portlanders feel so lucky to live here: this hilltop park complex practically right in the middle of town features a network of wilderness trails linking a huge range of family-friendly things to see and do, not to mention postcard-quality views in all directions. This is Washington Park, the Southwest Portland companion to the adjoining (and somewhat wilder) Forest Park, an awesome 5,000-acre forested woodland that occupies a large part of Northwest Portland. Best of all, Washington Park is easy to get to: just hop on MAX Light Rail, take an elevator up to the surface, and you're standing in the midst of a handful of attractions, including several good museums and the Oregon Zoo. From there it's a short hike along softly winding forest paths to reach a pair of beautifully sculpted gardens. You'll want to bring snacks or a picnic for this walk, if only because you'll have an excuse to linger.

● Start at the Washington Park MAX Station, which is 260 feet underground. An elevator takes you up to surface level, more or less in the parking lot of the zoo.

● The Oregon Zoo has been in its current location since the late 1950s. It's probably most famous (at least locally) for being the home of Packy, the Asian elephant, part of the zoo's successful elephant-breeding program. The zoo also holds outdoor music concerts in the summer, and in December there are elaborate animatronic displays of holiday lights.

● From the zoo entrance, loop around the parking lot to reach the Portland Children's Museum. Recommended mostly for very little kids (under 5 years old or so), this is a safe place to turn your toddlers loose on a rainy day and let them run around from one hands-on creative-learning exhibit to the next—they can dig holes, buy groceries, fingerpaint, and so on. Kids can also attend vacation camps and group classes (in science, painting, yoga, and one that's all about making messes). The museum does get crammed on the weekends, and if you don't relish the idea of being in a room full of giggling, screaming, scampering tots, you might want to skip this one, but parents seem to love it.

● Continuing around the parking lot to your left, you'll come to the World Forestry Center, another kid-friendly museum, this one dedicated to understanding the value of forests in everyday life. Its exhibits cover forest use and preservation in various parts of the world, at levels that will interest kids but won't bore their parents. Outside stands a massive petrified stump from a giant Sequoia tree that's 5 million years old.

● Turn left on exiting the World Forestry Center, and follow the trail to the entrance of the Vietnam Veterans of Oregon Memorial. Dedicated in 1987, it lists the names of Oregon veterans who served in the war, as well as random events from around the state that were occurring at the same time. The memorial is situated in a shallow, grass-covered hollow; sections of the wall are distributed along a paved spiral sidewalk, which leads you gently up to the edge of the bowl and connects with the Wildwood Trail.

● Follow the spiral pathway from the memorial until it joins the Wildwood Trail. From here, you'll stay on the Wildwood to reach Hoyt Arboretum; the trail is well signposted, so it shouldn't be difficult to follow. Veer left at the spur trail to the arboretum (also clearly marked).

● Hoyt Arboretum is what it sounds like: a tree museum, spread out across 187 acres, showcasing 1,100 species of trees from around the world. The most casual appraisal makes it clear that this area is prime real estate, and it was originally intended for residential development. But before that could happen, civic leaders lobbied to preserve the land as a public space on which to conserve unusual or endangered tree species. In 1922, Multnomah County gave the land to the city of Portland for the park that became the arboretum. It's named after Ralph Warren Hoyt, one of the county commissioners who pushed to have it established. If time and energy allow, the trails winding through the arboretum are worth exploring on your own—the trees make especially vivid scenery in fall and spring.

- Backtrack from the arboretum entrance to return to the Wildwood Trail, and continue along the trail in the same direction you were heading before. The trail through this section of forest makes a number of switchbacks, and there are a few intersections with other trails, but it's well marked. After about 1.7 miles, on some of the switchbacks you should be able to catch the occasional glimpse of the Japanese Garden below you.

- In just under 2 miles you'll come to a spur trail off to the right that leads to the Japanese Garden. Established as part of Portland's sister-city relationship with Sapporo, Japan, the garden opened in 1967. It has five parts: the Strolling Pond Garden, the Tea Garden, the Natural Garden, the Flat Garden, and the Sand and Stone Garden. A tea house occasionally hosts formal tea ceremonies. An incredibly pretty, calming place, It's best on an overcast day (not difficult to achieve in Portland), when the lush green ferns and stone sculptures seem to glow. Tours are available daily; check the website for details.

- Exit the garden and cross the large parking lot at SW Kingston Ave. to enter the International Rose Test Garden. You'll recognize it from the millions of postcard snapshots that have been taken from here. The rose garden, like the rest of Washington Park, is a great place to wander idly, sniffing and looking at the unbelievable variety of roses in their tidy arrangements. There are supposedly 9,525 rose bushes here, representing 610 different types. This is also (understandably) a popular wedding spot. The garden is maintained by the Portland Rose Society, a nonprofit that has been around since the 1800s; it was established by the Pittock family, they of the mansion just over the next ridge, in Forest Park. (You can get a closer look at the Pittock Mansion on Walk 7: Forest Park). As you wander, don't miss the Frank L. Beach Memorial Fountain, designed by Lee Kelly in 1974 in honor of the man who gave Portland its "City of Roses" nickname.

POINTS OF INTEREST (START TO FINISH)

Oregon Zoo oregonzoo.org, 4001 SW Canyon Rd., 503-226-1561

Portland Children's Museum portlandcm.org, 4015 SW Canyon Rd., 503-223-6500

World Forestry Center worldforestry.org, 4033 SW Canyon Rd., 503-228-1367

Hoyt Arboretum hoytarboretum.org, 4000 SW Fairview Blvd., 503-865-8733

Japanese Garden japanesegarden.com, 611 SW Kingston Ave., 503-223-1321

International Rose Test Garden tinyurl.com/rosetestgarden, 850 SW Rose Garden Way, 503-823-3636

ROUTE SUMMARY

1. Start at the Washington Park MAX Station.
2. Circle the parking lot to the museum entrances.
3. From the World Forestry Center, follow the trail left to the Vietnam Veterans of Oregon Memorial.
4. Take the spiral path and merge onto the Wildwood Trail.
5. Turn left at the spur leading to the Hoyt Arboretum entrance.
6. Return from the arboretum entrance to the Wildwood Trail.
7. Turn right at the spur leading to the Japanese Garden entrance.
8. Cross the parking lot at SW Kingston Ave. to enter the International Rose Test Garden.

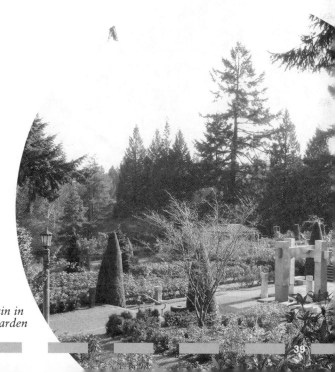

*The Frank L. Beach Memorial Fountain in
Washington Park's International Rose Test Garden*

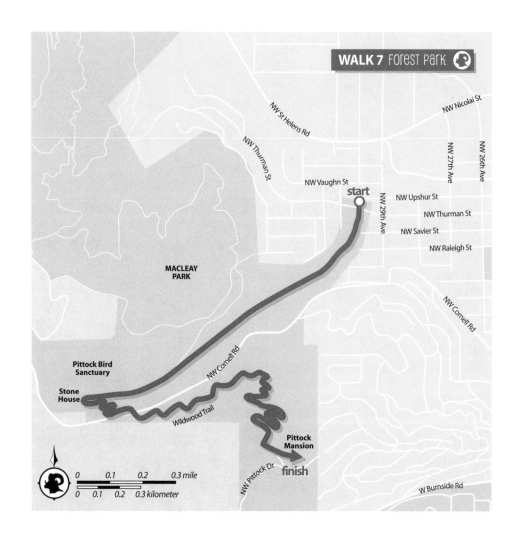

WALK 7 Forest Park

NW Nicolai St

NW St Helens Rd

NW Thurman St

NW 27th Ave

NW 26th Ave

NW Vaughn St

start

NW 29th Ave

NW Upshur St

NW Thurman St

NW Savier St

NW Raleigh St

MACLEAY
PARK

NW Cornell Rd

Pittock Bird
Sanctuary

Stone
House

NW Cornell Rd

Wildwood Trail

Pittock
Mansion

NW Pittock Dr

finish

W Burnside Rd

0   0.1   0.2   0.3 mile
0   0.1   0.2   0.3 kilometer

7 FOreST ParK: HOUSe ON THe HILL

BOUNDARIES: **NW 29th Ave., NW Upshur St., Forest Park, NW Pittock Dr.**
DISTANCE: **5 miles**
DIFFICULTY: **Moderate–strenuous**
PARKING: **Lot and street parking (both free)**
PUBLIC TRANSIT: **TriMet Bus 15 (numerous stops along NW Thurman St. near the park)**

It would be crazy not to recommend a walk in Forest Park, the largest and one of the richest urban parks in the country. It's essentially a huge wilderness right in Portland's backyard: some 5,000 acres of untouched forest laced with well-maintained trails of all lengths and levels. And many of its entry points are, like this trek to the historic Pittock Mansion, incredibly easy to get to from the city. It sounds cliché, but it's true: within minutes you can feel like you're miles away from anything resembling pavement, trekking through deep dark woods with sunlight filtering through a canopy of trees. (Or, perhaps more realistic, a faint mist hanging in the gray air—but even bad weather looks pretty in the woods.) This hike's accessibility makes it a popular choice, so it can get a little busy on weekends; go early in the morning or late in the afternoon to avoid any crowds. But even on a crowded day, it's well worth sharing the trail to reach those incredible views at the top.

- Start at the Lower Macleay Trailhead, where you'll find a small parking lot, restrooms, and a picnic table or two. Find it by following NW Thurman St. to 29th Ave., then going down the hill and turning left on Upshur St. (signs can be a little tricky to spot).

- From the parking lot, walk under the Thurman Street Bridge toward the red sculptures where the trail begins. You'll see a series of crumbling wooden structures on the left—this is where Balch Creek (which you'll follow for much of the walk) heads underground for a few miles on its way to the river. Balch Creek is named for Danford Balch, an early Oregon settler with quite a story. Balch and his family settled on 350 acres near Portland in 1850. In 1858, Balch's 16-year-old daughter, Anna, ran off with a ranch hand who went by the Gothic-literary name of Mortimer Stump (really). This did not go over well with old Danford. During the ensuing negotiations, tempers may have flared, and Danford Balch "accidentally" shot and killed Mortimer Stump. And that's how Balch became the first man sentenced to death and executed

Back Story: Pittock Mansion

Though it doesn't look quite like what we typically imagine a pioneer home to be, Pittock Mansion is, in a way, a pioneer home, if a very decadent and sophisticated one. It was built for Henry and Georgiana Pittock, who traveled here from Pennsylvania along the Oregon Trail and lived in the mansion from 1914 to 1919. But this wasn't exactly their "starter" home.

Henry Pittock, born in England, arrived in Portland at age 19 in 1853, completely broke. At the time Portland had a population of about 1,500 people. Henry got a job at the then weekly *Oregonian* newspaper and slowly began to work his way up the paper's chain of command. Seven years later, he bought the whole enterprise and turned it into a daily. That same year, Henry met and married Georgiana Martin Burton, who'd arrived from Missouri with her parents a year after he had. When they married, she was only 15 years old. The couple quickly became socialites and civic leaders, participating in the annual Rose Festival parade, forming relief organizations for children in need and for working women, and so on. They had six kids and built up a wide range of business interests. In 1909 they started planning and designing their house on the hill. By the time they moved into the mansion, Georgiana was 68 and Henry was 80. Georgiana died in 1918 and Henry in 1919. The house has been owned by the city of Portland since 1964 and was opened to the public the following year.

in Oregon (by hanging, in 1859). No word on how things turned out for his poor daughter.

- At the second wooden bridge, peek over the railing into the pool—you can usually catch sight of some cutthroat trout hiding there. And if you've got a keen eye, somewhere along the trail you might spot an owl lurking in the branches overhead.

- In just under a mile, you'll reach the Stone House, a perfect little moss-covered gray stone cottage. It was built by the Works Progress Administration as a public restroom, believe it or not, and served as such until 1962, when a huge storm destroyed the plumbing system and the park service decided it would cost too much to fix. Note the sawed-off slices of log arrayed around the trail, and feel free to take a load off for a while if you're so inclined.

- At the Stone House, the trail you're on divides—continue straight along the Wildwood Trail rather than turning right to go up the hill.

- About half a mile later, you'll cross Cornell Rd. at a crosswalk—be very careful, as this section of road is the fun, curvy sort that tempts drivers to think they're guesting on *Top Gear.* Continue uphill on the Wildwood Trail, along a fairly steep series of switch-backs. At a couple of places, the trail crosses the Upper Macleay Trail, but signs are clearly marked; just stay on the Wildwood, and any time you're in doubt, go uphill rather than down.

- You'll come out at the parking lot of the impressive Pittock Mansion. Completed in 1914, it was the home of Henry Pittock and his wife, Georgiana. The Pittocks arrived via the Oregon Trail, and Henry started work as a typesetter at the local paper. He worked his way up and eventually bought the newspaper, which he transformed into the daily *Oregonian.* You can take a tour of the mansion's interior ($8.50 per person), but it's nice enough (and free) just wandering the grounds, appreciating the sur-rounding gardens and taking in the awesome views, including Mt. Hood and, on a clear day, Mt. St. Helens and three other peaks. If it's nice out, eat your lunch on the front lawn of the mansion.

- Return to the parking lot the same way or, for something different, take a right onto the Upper Macleay Trail on your way down; it links back up with the Wildwood just above the Cornell Rd. crossing.

POINTS OF INTEREST (START TO FINISH)

Pittock Mansion pittockmansion.org, 3229 NW Pittock Dr., 503-823-3623

rouTe summary

1. From NW Thurman St., take NW 29th Ave. to NW Upshur St., and turn left to reach the Lower Macleay Trailhead.

2. At the Stone House, continue straight on the Wildwood Trail.

3. Cross Cornell Rd., staying on the Wildwood Trail.

4. Route ends at Pittock Mansion.

5. Return the way you came, or take a right onto the Upper Macleay Trail for a different route.

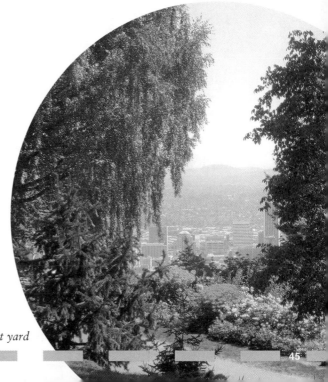

Downtown viewed from the Pittock Mansion's front yard

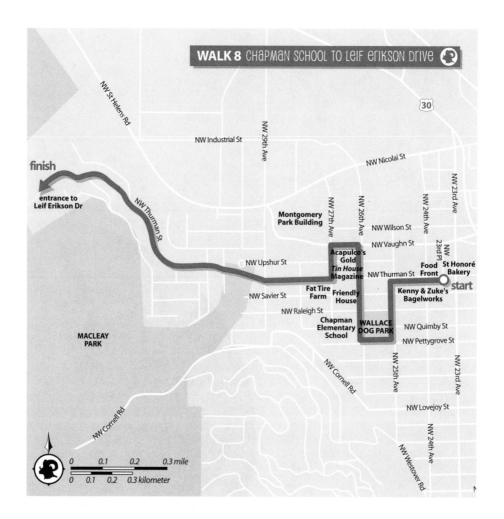

NW St Helens Rd

NW Industrial St

NW 29th Ave

30

NW Nicolai St

NW 23rd Ave

finish

NW 24th Ave

entrance to
Leif Erikson Dr

NW Thurman St

Montgomery
Park Building

NW 27th Ave

NW 26th Ave

NW Wilson St

NW Vaughn St

NW
23rd Pl

NW Upshur St

Acapulco's
Gold
Tin House
Magazine

NW Thurman St

Food
Front

St Honoré
Bakery

Fat Tire
Farm

Friendly
House

Kenny & Zuke's
Bagelworks

start

NW Savier St

NW Raleigh St

Chapman
Elementary
School

WALLACE
DOG PARK

NW Quimby St

NW Pettygrove St

MACLEAY
PARK

NW Cornell Rd

NW 25th Ave

NW 23rd Ave

NW Cornell Rd

NW Lovejoy St

NW 24th Ave

NW Westover Rd

| 0 | 0.1 | 0.2 | 0.3 mile |
| 0 | 0.1 | 0.2 | 0.3 kilometer |

8 Chapman School to Leif Erikson Drive: Swift Work

BOUNDARIES: **NW Vaughn St., NW 23rd Ave., NW Overton St., NW Cornell Rd., Forest Park**
DISTANCE: **2 miles, with option for longer hike**
DIFFICULTY: **Easy, with option for strenuous**
PARKING: **Free on street**
PUBLIC TRANSIT: **TriMet Bus 15 (NW 25th Ave. and Thurman St.)**

This walk, in an out-of-the-way little pocket of Portland, gives you the option for a longer hike into the forest at the end, depending on your stamina, interest, and fitness level. During late summer and fall, the route includes one of the city's most otherworldly and fascinating phenomena: the swooping and swirling bedtime rituals of the flock of Vaux's swifts that roost at Chapman Elementary School. (You can watch them most evenings from late August through September, depending on the weather and the restlessness of the birds. Until you've seen it, it's hard to appreciate what a cool thing this is, but trust us, it's worth the effort.)

Any time of year, this is a part of Northwest Portland that may not get much press but rewards exploration; one could describe it as "polished industrial." Springing up along Thurman and Upshur Streets are the offices of creative-class types—graphic designers, architects, photographers, and video-production workers—mixed in with the comfortably established residential neighborhood full of old leafy trees, wooden bungalows, and shiny new apartment buildings. Looming over all of this is the landmark Montgomery Park office building, whose red-neon sign is visible from most parts of Portland. The proximity of regular folks, creative industrial workers, and untamed forest makes this area an appealing section of town to wander around in.

● **Start at the corner of NW 23rd Pl. (not 23rd Ave.) and Thurman St., where you have no fewer than three fine choices for loading up on picnic supplies: St. Honoré Bakery, home of authentic French-style sandwiches and achingly beautiful pastries; Food Front Cooperative Grocery, a community-owned market of almost *Portlandia*-level earnestness, with organic produce and a gourmet deli; and Kenny & Zuke's**

Bagelworks, formerly Sandwichworks, where despite the name change you can still get some of the deli's famous hero sandwiches and grinders.

● Having stocked up on edibles, head up NW Thurman St. to NW 25th Ave. and turn left. In two blocks you'll reach the corner of the Wallace Dog Park, which you'll either love or hate depending on your canine-friendliness. (It's not just for dogs, of course, but they are a noticeable presence.) You can make your way diagonally across the park or walk its perimeter, along 25th Ave., then turn right on NW Pettygrove St.

● Chapman Elementary School and its surrounding lawn are a popular destination in late summer and early fall, when a huge flock of Vaux's swifts roosts here and preps for the long migratory trip to Central America. Anywhere from 2,000 to 7,000 of the birds bed down for the night in the school's chimney, and about an hour before sunset they start swirling and swooping around the place in a massive, billowing cloud. It's hard to imagine they can possibly all fit inside the chimney, but they seem to have it figured out. The maneuvering flock is really impressive to watch; grab a spot on the lawn and see for yourself. Local Audubon Society volunteers are usually around to answer any questions you might have about the birds.

● Cross the schoolyard to the right (east) and turn left on NW 26th Ave. At the corner of NW 26th and Thurman you'll see the Friendly House, originally the Marshall Street Community Center, founded by the Presbyterian church in 1926. (It has been called the Friendly House since 1930.) It's a nonprofit social services organization whose role in the community took shape early on, when volunteers here helped families get through the economic struggles of the Great Depression. These days, the Friendly House looks out in particular for underserved populations, including LGBT senior citizens and the kids of homeless families. There's also a wide range of workshops and classes for adults (for example, art therapy for people recovering from domestic abuse, yoga for senior citizens, and fitness for people with mobility issues), as well as camps, field trips, and preschool and after-school programs for kids. The mosaic-tile sculpture out front was designed by Lynn Takata and put together by Friendly House volunteers and supporters in 2011.

● Crossing NW Thurman St., notice the tall, skinny, metallic bungalow at the corner. This is the home of *Tin House* magazine's Portland headquarters. (There are also offices in Brooklyn.) Yep, it's an actual tin house! If you haven't encountered the *Tin House* literary mag before, make a point of picking up the latest issue. There's also a newish book-publishing division, with a roster of critically acclaimed indie successes recently, including Alexis Smith's *Glaciers* and Christopher Beha's *What Happened to Sophie Wilder.* The publisher also holds an annual weeklong writers workshop each summer at Portland's Reed College campus, with readings and lectures that are open to the public.

● At NW Vaughn St., turn left to find the rough-around-the-edges Mexican restaurant and bar Acapulco's Gold. The place is famous for its awesome margaritas and not-that-great-but-really-cheap food. One side is a lunch counter, the other side a dark and punked-out bar, and both are crammed with kitsch and murals.

● Walking up NW Vaughn St. toward 27th Ave., you'll be able to see the Montgomery Park Building and its huge red sign (lit up sort of fetchingly at night). Built in 1920, the structure was once part of Montgomery Ward's catalog business, part of the company's efforts to expand its mail-order markets westward, into the Pacific Northwest, Alaska, and Hawaii. At the time it was the largest commercial building in Portland (even before it was expanded in 1936). It was built on the site of the 1905 Lewis and Clark Centennial Exposition (see Back Story, next page). Montgomery Ward was here until the mid-1980s, when the company closed and sold the warehouse. Bought and renovated by the Naito family (who were reportedly pleased that they only had to change the *W* and the *D* in the sign), it now houses office buildings and trade-show space.

● Turn left on NW 27th Ave. for a block, then right onto NW Thurman St. At the corner is Fat Tire Farm, one of the earliest and best-liked bicycle shops in town. You can rent a mountain bike here to go exploring in Forest Park, as well as pick up maps and get all kinds of advice on bike trails, commuting, repairs, and the bicycle community in Portland. Unlike a few other shops in town, the staff here don't make you feel like an idiot if you don't already happen to be an expert cyclist—it's a good place to ask questions and find help without being intimidated.

● Continue along NW Thurman St. through increasingly quiet blocks. At NW 29th Ave. you'll cross the bridge over Macleay Park, with stairs allowing you to drop down to

BACK STORY: 1905 LEWIS AND CLARK CENTENNIAL EXPOSITION

The summer and early fall of 1905 saw Portland's first and only world's fair, the Lewis and Clark Centennial Expo. Millions of people showed up, and many of them stayed; the city's population doubled in the next five years. World's fairs in general were a chance for people to see the very newest and most exciting advancements in architecture, science, technology, and ideas. Twenty-one countries participated in the Lewis and Clark Expo, each with an elaborately decorated pavilion meant to display its glorious bounty. Often the pavilions themselves *were* the display, as in the case of the Forest Building, which was made of huge Douglas-fir logs, bark and all, and meant to represent the potential of the logging industry in the Pacific Northwest. (It stayed up and in use until a fire destroyed it in 1964.) Many of the structures were later taken apart and moved to other parts of town when the Expo ended—for instance, the McMenamins theater pub in St. Johns and its original dome (see Walk 25: St. Johns and Cathedral Park for details).

the little park and picnic area where the Lower Macleay Trail begins (and where you could also link up with Walk 7: Forest Park). Otherwise, or after a picnic break, forge ahead on NW Thurman St. as it winds its way uphill and the houses and yards grow ever more attractive. At the end of the curvy street, you'll come to a gateway that marks the entrance to NW Leif Erikson Dr. (Sometimes also called Leif Erikson Trail, it was named Hillside Dr. until 1933, when the local Sons of Norway lobbied to change the name in honor of the Norwegian explorer.) This trail is a nice wide dirt-and-gravel road that stretches 11 miles into Forest Park; it's a favorite among runners and bicyclists. We'll turn you loose here to decide for yourself how far you feel like going. (This trail is also a fine entry point for more-extensive hikes throughout Forest Park, but you'll definitely want to have a good map on hand.)

● To return to the starting point, simply reverse course and follow NW Thurman St. to NW 23rd Pl. Or hop Bus 15 back; you can catch it at NW Gordon St.

POINTS OF INTEREST (START TO FINISH)

St. Honoré Bakery sainthonorebakery.com, 2335 NW Thurman St., 503-445-4342

Food Front Cooperative Grocery foodfront.coop, 2375 NW Thurman St., 503-222-5658

Kenny & Zuke's Bagelworks kzbagelworks.com, 2376 NW Thurman St., 503-954-1737

Friendly House friendlyhouseinc.org, 1737 NW 26th Ave., 503-228-4391

Tin House Magazine tinhouse.com, 2617 NW Thurman St.

Acapulco's Gold 2608–10 NW Vaughn St., 503-220-0283

Fat Tire Farm fattirefarm.com, 2714 NW Thurman St., 503-222-3276

ROUTE SUMMARY

1. Start at NW 23rd Pl. and Thurman St.
2. Follow NW Thurman St. to NW 25th Ave.; turn left.
3. Turn right on NW Pettygrove St..
4. Cross the schoolyard and turn left on NW 26th Ave.
5. Turn left on NW Vaughn St.
6. Turn left on NW 27th Ave.
7. Turn right on NW Thurman St.
8. Follow Thurman St. to gateway at start of NW Leif Erikson Dr.

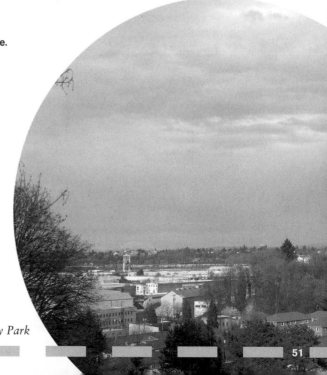

View from the Thurman Street Bridge over Macleay Park

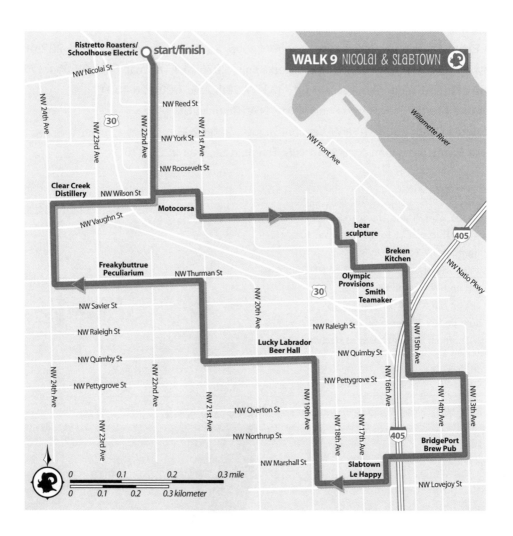

Ristretto Roasters/
Schoolhouse Electric ○ start/finish

WALK 9 Nicolai & Slabtown ◯

NW Nicolai St

NW Reed St

NW 24th Ave

30

NW 23rd Ave

NW 22nd Ave

NW 21st Ave

NW York St

NW Front Ave

Willamette River

NW Roosevelt St

Clear Creek
Distillery   NW Wilson St

Motocorsa

bear
sculpture

NW Vaughn St

405

Breken
Kitchen

NW Natio Pkwy

Freakybuttrue
Peculiarium   NW Thurman St

Olympic
Provisions
Smith
Teamaker

30

NW Savier St

NW 20th Ave

NW 15th Ave

NW Raleigh St

NW Raleigh St

Lucky Labrador
Beer Hall

NW Quimby St

NW Quimby St

NW 16th Ave

NW 24th Ave

NW 22nd Ave

NW Pettygrove St

NW Pettygrove St

NW 14th Ave

NW 13th Ave

NW 21st Ave

NW 19th Ave

NW Overton St

NW 23rd Ave

NW 18th Ave

NW 17th Ave

405

BridgePort
Brew Pub

NW Northrup St

NW Marshall St

Slabtown
Le Happy

NW Lovejoy St

0   0.1   0.2   0.3 mile

0   0.1   0.2   0.3 kilometer

9 NICOLaI aND SLaBTOWN: rOUGH aND reaDY

BOUNDARIES: **NW Front Ave., NW Nicolai St., NW 24th Ave., NW Lovejoy St.**
DISTANCE: **3 miles**
DIFFICULTY: **Easy**
PARKING: **Free on street; small lot near start/finish**
PUBLIC TRANSIT: **TriMet Bus 16 (NW Front Ave. and Nicolai St.)**

This walk covers an odd little slice of Portland between the posh NW 23rd and 21st Avenues and the river, with the hard-core Industrial Northwest neighborhood to the north. It's a funky, gritty, and not always attractive mix of freight containers and warehouses, coffee laboratories and mysterious museums. It's also one of the few parts of Portland that still feels refreshingly rough around the edges, even as indicators of sophistication (Italian motorcycles, Italian-style coffee) gradually venture in.

The neighborhood overall is poised to see massive and dramatic changes, thanks to freight company Con-way's plans to develop 18 acres in the area that are currently occupied by endless parking lots and the occasional colorless warehouse. (Con-way currently employs some 750 people in the offices on its property here.) The plans for development, to which the city has just recently given final approval, include a revision of one particularly snarly intersection (the trickiest part of the plans, and the reason it took so long for the project to win city approval), plus 2,500 homes, some parks, a library, and a mix of retail, including an upmarket grocery store. It's unclear how quickly the development will happen, but when it does, this neighborhood will be utterly transformed. Stay tuned!

● **Start your walk with some high-grade caffeine at Ristretto Roasters, a gorgeous coffee shop inside the restored Schoolhouse Electric & Supply Co. warehouse building at NW Nicolai St. and 21st Ave. You can get a pour-over and, at the same time, an aesthetically pleasing object lesson in what's been happening recently, architecture-wise, in the industrial and formerly industrial parts of Northwest Portland. (Schoolhouse Electric itself is pretty cool, too—browse its impressively restored 5,000-square-foot showroom for beautifully designed and redesigned lighting, luxurious textiles, rescued and repurposed furniture, hardware, fixtures, and more.)**

- Cross NW Nicolai St. and continue straight along NW 22nd Ave. past empty shipping containers and random industrial equipment until you get to NW Wilson St. Take a left on Wilson (although you may want to stop in at Motocorsa for a peek at some very shiny Italian motorcycles—it's a Ducati dealership, and quite fancy inside). From Wilson, hang a right onto NW 21st Ave., then a left onto NW Vaughn St. This might not be the most scenic part of Portland, but it's interesting from a behind-the-scenes point of view.

- Follow Vaughn as it bends to the right; turn left at NW Upshur St., and don't miss the scary metal sculpture of an angry bear (made of gears and metal scraps) in front of Castaways nightclub. From here you also have a cool view of the underside of the Fremont Bridge.

- Take a right at NW 17th Ave., then a left onto NW Thurman St. You can stop here to pick up some charcuterie at Olympic Provisions, or just admire the pretty facade of the Smith Teamaker building next door.

- Continue along NW Thurman St. to the funky-looking Triangle Building, where you can get a hearty meal worthy of a stevedore at Breken Kitchen. Take a right onto NW 15th Ave., and follow it underneath the highway bridges. Continue along 15th, then turn left onto NW Pettygrove St. and right onto NW 13th Ave. At the corner of NW 13th and Marshall St. is the first of Portland's major craft-beer joints, BridgePort Brew Pub (their winter seasonal brew, Ebenezer Ale, is one of our favorites). Though the place has fancied itself up a bit since its no-frills beer-and-pizza early days, hopheads and beer historians will find it well worth a pilgrimage.

- Take a right to walk up NW Marshall St., crossing underneath the highway bridges again. This area is loosely known as Slabtown—named for the huge slabs of lumber once used for heat and produced in nearby lumber mills. A more recent highlight of the neighborhood is also called Slabtown—but it's a rock club, a great local dive with live garage rock, cheap food, and pinball. It's at the corner of NW 16th Ave. and Marshall St. If that's not quite your scene, turn left on NW 16th and one door over you'll find Le Happy, a sweet little crêperie.

- From NW 16th Ave., take a right on NW Lovejoy St. and another right on NW 19th Ave. At NW Quimby St., go left. You'll pass Lucky Labrador Beer Hall, one of several locations for this brewery whose trademark is that people can bring their dogs along while they have a pint.

- Continue up NW Quimby and take a right on NW 21st Ave. The parking lot you're walking past is part of the planned development by Con-way Freight, which is certain to change the character of this neighborhood pretty substantially. (It's a BIG parking lot.)

- Turn left on NW Thurman St. In the tall, hot-pink building on your left—you can't miss it—is the Freakybuttrue Peculiarium, a little shop that looks like any old convenience store at first but gets weird once you step inside. A small museum of goofy oddities takes up most of the room; it's silly but fun. (Just don't get your neck stuck in the alien-autopsy display.)

- From NW Thurman St., take a right on NW 24th Ave. At NW 24th and Wilson St. you'll find Clear Creek Distillery, makers of a famous pear brandy made with the pear grown inside the bottle, among other things. Tours are available; check online for schedules.

- Turn right on NW Wilson St. and follow it back to the original route, turning left at NW 22nd Ave. to return to the starting point.

POINTS OF INTEREST (START TO FINISH)

Ristretto Roasters ristrettoroasters.com, 2181 NW Nicolai St., 503-227-2866

Schoolhouse Electric & Supply Co. schoolhouseelectric.com, 2181 NW Nicolai St., 503-230-7113

Olympic Provisions olympicprovisions.com, 1632 NW Thurman St., 503-894-8136

Breken Kitchen brekenkitchen.com, 1800 NW 16th Ave., 503-841-6359

BridgePort Brew Pub bridgeportbrew.com, 1313 NW Marshall St., 503-241-3612

Slabtown slabtownbar.net, 1033 NW 16th Ave., 971-229-1455

Le Happy lehappy.com, 1011 NW 16th Ave., 503-226-1258

Lucky Labrador Beer Hall luckylab.com, 1945 NW Quimby St., 503-517-4352

Freakybuttrue Peculiarium peculiarium.com, 2234 NW Thurman St.

Clear Creek Distillery clearcreekdistillery.com, 2389 NW Wilson St., 503-248-9470

route summary

1. Start at NW Nicolai St. and 21st Ave.
2. Cross Nicolai, continue to NW 22nd Ave., and turn left on NW Wilson St.
3. Turn right on NW 21st Ave.
4. Turn left on NW Vaughn St.
5. Turn left on NW Upshur St.
6. Turn right on NW 17th Ave.
7. Turn left on NW Thurman St.
8. Turn right on NW 15th Ave.
9. Turn left onto NW Pettygrove St.
10. Turn right on NW 13th Ave.
11. Turn right on NW Marshall St.
12. Turn left on 16th Ave.
13. Turn right on Lovejoy St.
14. Turn right on 19th Ave.
15. Turn left on Quimby St.
16. Turn right on 21st Ave.
17. Turn left on Thurman St.
18. Turn right on 24th Ave.
19. Turn right on Wilson St.
20. Turn left on 22nd Ave.

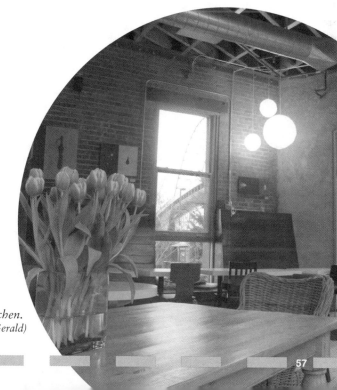

Refuel at Breken Kitchen.
(Photo courtesy of Paul Gerald)

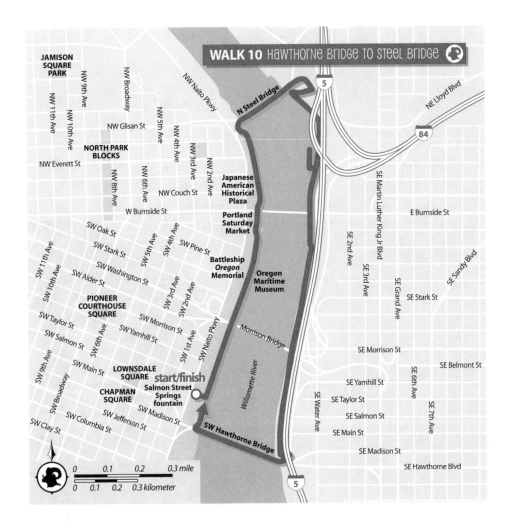

JAMISON
SQUARE
PARK

NW 9th Ave

NW Broadway

NW Naito Pkwy

N Steel Bridge

NW 11th Ave

NW 10th Ave

NW 5th Ave

NW 4th Ave

NW Glisan St

NORTH PARK
BLOCKS

NW Everett St

NW 8th Ave

NW 6th Ave

NW 3rd Ave

NW 2nd Ave

NW Couch St

Japanese
American
Historical
Plaza

W Burnside St

Portland
Saturday
Market

SW Oak St

SW Stark St

SW 5th Ave

SW 4th Ave

SW Pine St

Battleship
Oregon
Memorial

SW Washington St

SW Alder St

SW 11th Ave

SW 10th Ave

SW 3rd Ave

SW 2nd Ave

Oregon
Maritime
Museum

PIONEER
COURTHOUSE
SQUARE

SW Taylor St

SW 6th Ave

SW Morrison St

SW Yamhill St

SW 1st Ave

SW Naito Pkwy

SW Salmon St

Morrison Bridge

SW 9th Ave

SW Main St

LOWNSDALE
SQUARE

SW Broadway

start/finish

Salmon Street
Springs
fountain

Willamette River

CHAPMAN
SQUARE

SW Columbia St

SW Jefferson St

SW Madison St

SW Clay St

SW Hawthorne Bridge

5

84

NE Lloyd Blvd

SE Martin Luther King Jr Blvd

E Burnside St

SE 2nd Ave

SE 3rd Ave

SE Grand Ave

SE Stark St

SE Sandy Blvd

SE Morrison St

SE Belmont St

SE Yamhill St

SE 6th Ave

SE 7th Ave

SE Taylor St

SE Salmon St

SE Water Ave

SE Main St

SE Madison St

SE Hawthorne Blvd

5

0   0.1   0.2   0.3 mile

0   0.1   0.2   0.3 kilometer

10 HawtHorne Bridge to Steel Bridge: ring around the river

BOUNDARIES: **Steel Bridge, SW Front Ave., Hawthorne Bridge, I-5**
DISTANCE: **3 miles**
DIFFICULTY: **Easy**
PARKING: **Free street parking, metered near Hawthorne side of Eastbank Esplanade**
PUBLIC TRANSIT: **TriMet Buses 4, 10, and 14 (SW Main St. and 2nd Ave.); MAX Blue and Red Lines (Yamhill District Station)**

This is an easy, pleasant (in nice weather) waterfront loop walk that includes two of Portland's more noteworthy, character-defining civic projects, both of which exist mainly thanks to the progressive vision of city leaders who were intent on preserving the city's reputation for pedestrian-friendly travel and that old magazine favorite, "livability." Along with great views and fresh air, this walk provides some tangible examples of that often-vague concept, in the form of the Eastbank Esplanade and Waterfront Park. It's also a great way to get a feel for Portland's overall layout, the difference in character between the east side and the west side of the Willamette River, and the importance of bridges and the Willamette River in the city's general atmosphere.

- Start at the Salmon Street Springs fountain, at the foot of SW Salmon St. near the riverfront. Busy with frolicking toddlers and teens all summer long, the fountain is a familiar and oft-photographed city landmark, as well as a handy meeting point. Fun fact: it has 185 water jets, whose three shifting patterns are controlled by a computer stored underground.

- From the fountain, head toward the river and left along the seawall. The original version of this wall was built in the 1920s to keep the Willamette River from flooding downtown every year. What is now Tom McCall Waterfront Park was a major traffic thoroughfare for years, until the opening of the Marquam Bridge and I-5 provided a more efficient alternative. In the late 1960s, then-Gov. Tom McCall started looking at plans to replace the outdated road (called Harbor Dr.) with some type of public space. (One suggestion, which in retrospect seems borderline-insane, was to make

Harbor Dr. even wider.) The park was finished and dedicated in 1978 (and was officially named after McCall in 1984). A tremendously popular place to hang out year-round, it's typically buzzing with a mix of walkers, runners, inline skaters, napping or lunching office workers, homeless people, tourists, and various festivals. (It's the main location of the annual Rose Festival, for instance, as well as a bunch of warm-weather beer- and food-themed extravaganzas.) In 2012 the American Planning Association called it one of the 10 Great Public Spaces, and it's hard to argue with that.

- Heading farther north along the waterfront, you'll come to an incongruous white pillar sticking out of the ground. This is the Battleship *Oregon* Memorial, which commemorates a ship from the late 1800s known as the "Bulldog of the U.S. Navy"; a time capsule in its base is due to be opened in 2076.

- Just across the park, at the foot of SW Pine St., is the sternwheeler *Portland*. The ship has been semiretired and is now home to the Oregon Maritime Museum, a kid-friendly favorite among Portland's tourist activities. It usually stays moored but recently has been taken out on occasional summertime exhibition trips. The sternwheeler is the last steam-powered tugboat built and operated in the US; a tour of the ship is included as part of a visit to the Maritime Museum.

- Farther along the waterfront, the wide, partly covered plaza that stretches from beneath the Burnside Bridge is the site of Portland's ever-expanding Saturday Market, a weekly outdoor arts and crafts and food bonanza that involves a satisfying amount of street theater and, naturally, elephant ears alongside its tie-dye clogs and vegan dreamcatchers. It runs every weekend (including Sundays, despite the name) from March through December.

- On the other side of the Burnside Bridge, at the foot of NW Couch St., is the Japanese American Historical Plaza. During World War II, Japanese Americans in the area were forced into internment camps; this plaza is dedicated to their memories, and artwork in the memorial garden portrays important moments from Japanese-American history.

- Continue along the waterfront path until you come to the Steel Bridge. Take the stairs up to the upper level (you can also stay on the lower level and cross that way; it's equally interesting either way, but the views are just slightly better from the top level). Opened in 1912, the Steel Bridge was built for the Union Pacific Railroad, and in choosing which level to take you've already discovered one of its unique characteristics: it has two decks that can move independently. The lower deck is designed for walkers, cyclists, and railroad traffic, while the upper level is for motorized traffic and light rail.

- At the far (east) end of the bridge, zigzag your way right, to ground level, to link with the Eastbank Esplanade.

Eastbank Esplanade, Portland's *other* long-and-skinny riverside greenway, is perhaps best loved for the views it provides of Tom McCall Waterfront Park. Which isn't to say it lacks its own charms. But its proximity to highways and the constraints of geography—it fits rather snugly into the thin space that has been allotted for it—mean there isn't much greenery to pretty up the path. It's kind of utilitarian, which doesn't bother the joggers and cyclists who use it one bit. Besides, the views across the river are glorious, and the esplanade is attractive in its own *Gattaca*-esque way. The walkway was dedicated to former Mayor Vera Katz (who fought for the park and is primarily responsible for its construction) in 2004. It's 1.5 miles long, extending from the Steel Bridge to the Hawthorne Bridge. The walkway is illuminated at night, which is particularly great during winter when it gets dark early (and light late). A 1,200-foot section floats out over the water, lending the esplanade a romantic, marina-like feel. It's also an environmental asset: part of the trail doubles as a water-treatment system, filtering runoff from I-5 before it gets to the river. Public art installations are found at several points along the trail—beneath the Morrison Bridge, look for *Echo Gate,* a copper sculpture meant to mirror downtown Portland's historic architecture. Another favorite is *Ghost Ship,* an impressive work in glass, copper, and steel.

- Follow the esplanade all the way to its end at the Hawthorne Bridge, winding your way up the circular path onto the bridge. The Hawthorne is the only vertical-lift bridge in North America that's older than the Steel Bridge. If you commute with any frequency between downtown and Southeast Portland, you may be convinced that the bridge is perpetually being raised, and in fact it does lift up around 200 times a month. Aside from making way for tall river traffic, the bridge needs to move at least once every 8 hours in order to keep its gears from sticking. (Don't worry—if you're walking across, you'll have plenty of warning before it goes up.) As you walk across

Back Story: Dr. James C. Hawthorne

If no one has yet written a historical novel about Hawthorne Boulevard's namesake, it's high time: Dr. James Hawthorne seems like a figure ripe for novelization, at least based on the bare factual outline of his life. A native of Pennsylvania, Hawthorne (1819–1881) spent several years working in medicine in California, where he was also elected to the state Senate. He moved to Portland in 1857 to run a facility for the mentally ill, and then in 1862 he took charge of the Oregon Hospital for the Insane, the state's first such institution (it occupied 200 acres around the intersection of SE Hawthorne Boulevard and 10th Avenue). Known as a caring, forward-thinking, and compassionate man, Hawthorne ran the asylum until he died, at which point there were somewhere around 500 inmates there. Hawthorne was married twice: his first wife, Emily Curry, died just a few weeks after they were married. In 1865 he married Mrs. E. C. Hite, from Sacramento, and they had three daughters, one of whom died in infancy.

Dr. Hawthorne is buried in Lone Fir Cemetery (see Walk 15: Stark-Belmont); according to the cemetery's website, some 132 of his patients are also buried there, though their graves are unmarked and the exact locations now uncertain. The patients were buried in the same part of the cemetery that was used for Portland's many Chinese workers during the 1890s, some of whom were later disinterred and repatriated for permanent burial in China. Metro, the regional government in charge of Lone Fir maintenance and operation, has planned a memorial garden to commemorate the sad histories of the asylum patients and the Chinese workers who were buried here. (For more about the plan, visit Metro's website, **tinyurl.com/lonefirmemorial.**)

the seams in the panels that form the pedestrian walkway, look down for a little dose of vertigo.

● As you come to the end of the bridge, turn right and descend the stairs to rejoin the Waterfront Park path and return to your starting point.

POINTS OF INTEREST (STArT TO FINISH)

Oregon Maritime Museum oregonmaritimemuseum.org, 115 SW Ash St., 503-224-7724

rOUTe SUMMArY

1. Start at the Salmon Street Springs fountain, at the foot of SW Salmon St.
2. Turn left at the Willamette River.
3. At the Steel Bridge, take a right to cross on the lower level, or climb the stairs to use the top deck.
4. Turn right at the end of the bridge to reach the Eastbank Esplanade.
5. Follow the esplanade onto the Hawthorne Bridge.
6. At the end of the Hawthorne Bridge, turn right and go down the stairs.

CONNECTING THE WALKS

Link with Walk 1: Old Town and Chinatown, Walk 12: Industrial Southeast, or Walk 14: Hawthorne Blvd. from various points along this route.

View of the river and the Steel Bridge from the Burnside Bridge

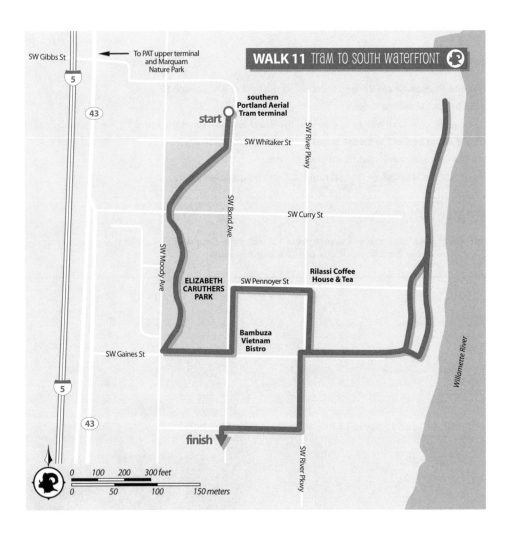

SW Gibbs St

← To PAT upper terminal and Marquam Nature Park

5

43

WALK 11 Tram to South Waterfront

southern
**Portland Aerial
Tram terminal**

start ○

SW Whitaker St

SW River Pkwy

SW Bond Ave

SW Curry St

**Rilassi Coffee
House & Tea**

SW Pennoyer St

**ELIZABETH
CARUTHERS
PARK**

SW Moody Ave

**Bambuza
Vietnam
Bistro**

SW Gaines St

5

43

finish ▼

SW River Pkwy

Willamette River

0   100   200   300 feet
0   50   100   150 meters

11 Tram to South Waterfront: The Sci-Fi Walk

BOUNDARIES: **Willamette River, SW Gibbs St., SW Abernethy St., SW 10th Ave.**
DISTANCE: **2 miles**
DIFFICULTY: **Easy (or moderate if you add a Marquam Trail hike)**
PARKING: **Metered, in OHSU lot**
PUBLIC TRANSIT: **TriMet Bus 8 (OHSU), tram, Portland Streetcar to downtown**

If you too grew up devouring unhealthy quantities of science-fiction paperbacks with garishly painted covers, you will automatically love the Portland Aerial Tram. Who cares if it's practical? *Look at it!* The tram makes Portland's skyline 50 times more awesome than before. Its other purpose, of course, is to carry people between Oregon Health & Science University (OHSU), perched high on the hillside, and the South Waterfront, a newly developed neighborhood in a previously industrial area alongside the river south of downtown. The South Waterfront development occupies a former "brown field"—land that was contaminated with the by-products of heavy industrial use, and which required a $20 million cleanup effort that has been going on since the 1990s. (A large portion of the industry that once occupied this area involved barge-building, and some of that is still going on; U.S. Navy ships were built here for World War II, and then dismantled here afterward.) The cleanup of the area is essentially wrapped up, and development continues—the location of this area makes it a potentially very exciting area for developers.

This walk takes us via the tram from OHSU's Marquam Hill location down through the South Waterfront neighborhood, with a bit of exploring on top of the hill first for those who are so inclined. If you're feeling even more ambitious, Metro (the regional government) maintains a linked network called the 4T Trail: it forms a loop that incorporates the Portland Streetcar, which connects to MAX Light Rail, which leads to the Wildwood Trail, which takes you to the tram (trail, tram, trolley, train = four Ts). Maps and guides are available online at **library.oregonmetro.gov/files/trailtramtrolleytrain.pdf.**

Note: Due to space constraints, our map begins at the south PAT terminal and does not show the upper PAT terminal or Marquam Nature Park. You can find maps of the park online at **fmnp.org** or at the Marquam Shelter, at the Marquam Trail entrance.

● Start at the upper terminal of the Portland Aerial Tram, in the OHSU Hospital complex. While you're up here, take advantage of the easy access to the wilderness trails through Marquam Nature Park, a 176-acre wilderness laced with around 5 miles of trails. To reach the closest trailhead, turn left along SW Sam Jackson Park Rd., past several OHSU buildings; then turn right on SW 9th Ave. and, tucked behind the motorcycle and scooter parking, you'll see the sign marking the start of Connor Trail. This path loops around toward the west and south to eventually meet up with the Marquam Trail, part of the regional 40-Mile Loop system (see Back Story: 40-Mile Loop, opposite), and is well worth a detour if you have the time and inclination.

● Retrace your steps back along SW Sam Jackson Park Rd. to reach the upper terminal of the Aerial Tram. Riding the tram costs $4 round-trip (unless you have a TriMet ticket already), and it runs about every 6 minutes most days. Aside from being adorable, the tram was also an audacious undertaking design-wise, and rather expensive. As with most such ambitious projects, its construction was not without detractors. Some neighbors (bafflingly!) felt that the tram would not aesthetically enhance the Portland skyline. Most of the criticism, though, was budgetary—especially after the projected cost of the tram doubled during the planning process. Some residents wondered if it was fair for taxpayers to foot part of the bill for a service that would be used primarily by OHSU students and staff. (The city's share of the total cost was 15%, or $8.5 million.) Ultimately, though, the project was approved, and the tram opened to the public in December 2006. It has carried more than 5 million riders so far. Its construction paved the way for development in the South Waterfront area, particularly by OHSU.

● The south terminal of the tram—the starting point of the map on page 64—is at OHSU's lower office building, near the north side of the South Waterfront development. (Adding to the whole cuteness factor, the lower lawn is "mowed" each year by three or four goats. *Aww.*) The popular Daily Cafe, inside the lower tram terminal, is a good option for refreshments in this neighborhood (so far there's not much else to choose from). Take SW Bond Ave. a block south to Elizabeth Caruthers Park. Cross the park diagonally to the corner of SW Moody Ave. and Curry St. Cross SW Curry St. to the next lot, a landscaped green space; walk across this to the corner of SW Gaines St. and Moody Ave. Turn left at Gaines St.

BaCK STOry: 40-MILe LOOP

If you spend any time on trails in the Portland area at all, you're likely to hear about the 40-Mile Loop metro-area trail system. This, as you might imagine, is a system of interconnected trails, some well established and others still in the planning stages. It includes the excellent Wildwood Trail through Forest Park, as well as bike-friendly urban corridors like the I-205 Path, Springwater Corridor, and Eastbank Esplanade. The "40-Mile" part of the name refers to city leaders' original conception of a regional trail network, an idea first dreamed up a century ago; when trail advocates revived the project in 1982, they called it the 40-Mile Loop in honor of that original vision.

These days the trail plan covers several cities and counties close to Portland, and the total mileage of the envisioned trail network is more like 950; the Multnomah County section alone incorporates some 30 parks and 140 miles of trail. For more details about the 40-Mile Loop, including maps of current and future trails, visit **40mileloop.org** (you can also get maps and information at Portland visitor centers).

● At SW Bond Ave., you'll come to one of the few dining options in this neighborhood so far: Bambuza Vietnam Bistro. (All the buildings are designed with retail and dining on the ground level, so eventually this will change.) You're basically in the heart of the development now; it's new enough and shiny enough to have a distinctly futuristic feel.

● Follow SW Bond St. for a block, then turn right at SW Pennoyer St. Where Pennoyer meets SW River Pkwy., there's another place to stop for a snack or a drink: Rilassi Coffee House & Tea. The corner is guarded by stone lions, echoed with enthusiasm inside the coffee shop, but the area outside still feels very angular and shiny. Turn right on River Pkwy., then left on SW Gaines St., which leads to a short pedestrian-only path along the riverfront. Follow the path to its end, take in the view across the water—you can see the Ross Island Bridge as well as Ross Island itself—then retrace your steps.

● At SW Gaines St. and River Pkwy., turn left, then take your first right up to SW Bond Ave., where you can catch a streetcar toward downtown.

POINTS OF INTEREST (START TO FINISH)

Marquam Nature Park fmnp.org, SW Sam Jackson Park Rd. and SW Marquam St.

Daily Cafe at the Tram dailycafe.net, 3355 SW Bond Ave., 503-224-9691

Bambuza Vietnam Bistro bambuza.com, 3682 SW Bond Ave., 503-206-6330

Rilassi Coffee House & Tea rilassicoffeehouse.com, 3580 SW River Pkwy., 503-467-7532

ROUTE SUMMARY

1. Start at the upper terminal of the Portland Aerial Tram.
2. Exit the tram's lower terminal.
3. Take SW Bond Ave. one block south, to Elizabeth Caruthers Park.
4. Cross the park diagonally to the corner of SW Curry St. and Moody Ave.
5. Cross SW Curry St. to the green space.
6. Cross the green space to the corner of SW Gaines St. and Moody Ave.
7. Turn left on SW Gaines St.
8. Turn left on SW Bond Ave.
9. Turn right on SW Pennoyer St.
10. Turn right on SW River Pkwy.
11. Turn left on SW Gaines St.
12. Follow the pedestrian path to its end, then retrace your steps.
13. Turn left on SW River Pkwy.
14. Take first right to reach SW Bond Ave.

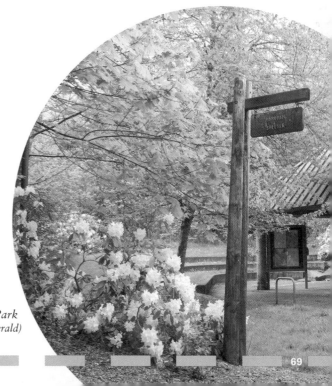

Marquam Nature Park
(Photo courtesy of Paul Gerald)

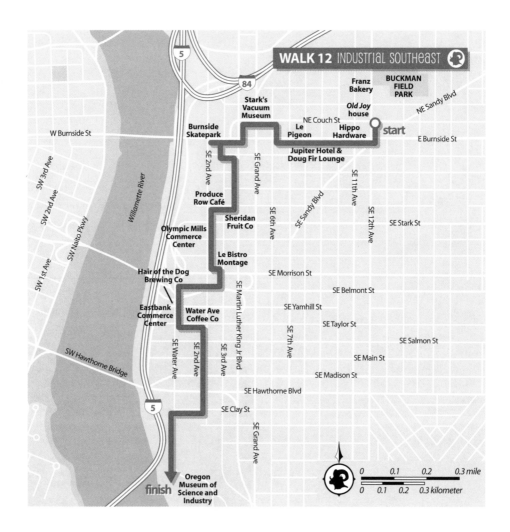

WALK 12 INDUSTRIAL SOUTHEAST

5

84

Franz Bakery

BUCKMAN FIELD PARK

NE Sandy Blvd

Stark's Vacuum Museum

Old Joy house

Burnside Skatepark

NE Couch St

Le Pigeon

Hippo Hardware

start

E Burnside St

W Burnside St

SW 3rd Ave

SW 2nd Ave

SE 2nd Ave

SE Grand Ave

Jupiter Hotel & Doug Fir Lounge

SE 11th Ave

SE 12th Ave

SE Stark St

Produce Row Café

SE 6th Ave

SE Sandy Blvd

Sheridan Fruit Co

Willamette River

SW Naito Pkwy

Olympic Mills Commerce Center

Le Bistro Montage

SE Morrison St

SE Belmont St

SW 1st Ave

Hair of the Dog Brewing Co

SE Yamhill St

SE Martin Luther King Jr Blvd

SE Taylor St

SE Salmon St

Eastbank Commerce Center

Water Ave Coffee Co

SE 7th Ave

SE Water Ave

SE 2nd Ave

SE 3rd Ave

SE Main St

SW Hawthorne Bridge

SE Madison St

SE Hawthorne Blvd

5

SE Clay St

SE Grand Ave

0   0.1   0.2   0.3 mile

0   0.1   0.2   0.3 kilometer

finish

Oregon Museum of Science and Industry

12 INDUSTRIAL SOUTHEAST: PRODUCE ROW

BOUNDARIES: **NE Couch St., SE 11th Ave., Willamette River, SE Division St.**
DISTANCE: **2.5 miles**
DIFFICULTY: **Easy**
PARKING: **Free on street, $3 in lot at OMSI**
PUBLIC TRANSIT: **TriMet Buses 4, 6, 10, and 14 at Hawthorne Bridge; Buses 12, 19, and 20 at E. Burnside St. and NE Sandy Blvd.**

An amorphous area sometimes called the Eastside Industrial or Southeast Warehouse District, sometimes Produce Row, this part of town is currently among the fastest-changing. Parts of it can still legitimately be described as gritty (and we mean that in a good way). This is partly by design: the Central Eastside Industrial Council, a nonprofit group that looks out for the neighborhood's business interests, has lobbied to keep housing out of the area, in order to preserve its cool working-class feel (and prevent it from turning into the Pearl District). But it's not all rail yards and storage units here. A neighborhood landmark, the Produce Row Café has recently been snazzed up with a total remodel, and a few other chic new dining and drinking establishments have helped amp up the sophistication level, ready or not.

- Start at the bus stop at NE Couch St. and 12th Ave. Movie nerds should pause and take a look down NE 12th Ave. to the right, where you'll spot a yellow-and-blue house you might recognize from director Kelly Reichardt's movie *Old Joy*. And beyond that you'll see a well-loved Portland icon: the gigantic rotating loaf of bread that designates Franz Bakery, whose intoxicating aroma you can also usually smell from here depending on the time of day.

- Turn left and head down NE 12th Ave., then cross E. Burnside St. and turn right. (This intersection is notoriously confusing and can be a little hairy—stay alert.) On the left is Hippo Hardware, an oddball hardware store and local landmark whose labyrinthine interior is a gold mine of old rusty hinges, Victorian doorknobs, weird lamps, skeleton keys, and all sorts of antique fixtures. Treasure hunt!

- Two blocks down on the left is the Jupiter Hotel and Doug Fir Lounge, a boutique hotel with attached 300-capacity live-music venue, bar, and restaurant whose design set (or at least embraced) all kinds of trends when it opened in 2004. The upstairs restaurant-bar is what you might imagine every building in Aspen or Vail will look like in the future: rustic but glittery, simultaneously posh and woodsy. The restrooms are paneled in gold-veined mirror—totally disorienting, but kind of fabulous. Downstairs, the music venue leans more toward the log-cabin feel, and regardless of your feelings about the Doug Fir as a whole, it's a great place to see bands you love: everyone sounds fantastic here. The attached Jupiter Hotel works a sort of *Jetsons*–IKEA minimalist design into a 1960s motor-inn shape, and the small art gallery in its front office has interesting exhibits that change monthly. Across the street, and in the next block, is a strip of funky little vintage-clothing shops, novelty shops, and galleries well worth poking around in.

- In the next block you'll find one of the most talked-about restaurants in a much-talked-about restaurant scene: the always-packed Le Pigeon, run by James Beard Award–winning chef Gabriel Rucker. It's a beautiful, smallish space with an open kitchen and a meat-heavy dinner menu.

- Continue down Burnside past a string of appealingly rock-and-roll bars to NE 6th Ave. Turn right on 6th, then left on NE Couch St. At the corner of Couch and NE Grand Ave. you'll find Stark's Vacuum Museum, a strange little space inside a retail vacuum-cleaner store—basically a hallway where some 300 models of vacuums from various points in history (starting in the 1800s) are stored. It's free to go in, have a look, and count your blessings.

- Go one block farther along NE Couch, then turn left onto NE Martin Luther King Jr. Blvd. for a block. Cross the street and turn right to walk along E. Burnside St., just underneath the bridge ramp. Here, tucked under the east end of the bridge, is the Burnside Skatepark, generally considered one of the best skate parks in the country and—even if you're not into skating—an inspiring community project.

Before about 1990, underneath the Burnside Bridge was not a place you'd ever want to go. But a handful of skater kids started reclaiming the area, gradually adding to the empty concrete square until it became the enclosed park it is now. This took over a decade, and the feat of the park's construction is amazing in itself, but the real victory is that Burnside Skatepark, though built without permission, eventually won tentative acceptance by city government as a public skate park.

• Retrace your steps up E. Burnside St. and take a right on SE 3rd Ave., then a left on SE Ankeny St., then a right onto SE Martin Luther King Jr. Blvd. At the corner of MLK and SE Oak St. you'll find the Sheridan Fruit Company, a small grocery store that has been owned and operated by the same family since 1946. The produce and the deli here are excellent.

• Follow SE Oak St. two blocks down to SE 2nd Ave., where you'll come to the neighborhood's longstanding namesake pub, Produce Row Café. This former working-man's beer bar and sandwich shop underwent a radical transformation not long ago. It was always comfy, but now it's also stylish, and the back patio has been covered to accommodate the long rainy season. Food options at the "old" ProRow consisted of a few types of legendarily enormous sandwiches; these days you can get *moules frites* and radicchio salad, too. One thing that hasn't changed, thank goodness, is the massive beer selection (now with whiskey!).

• From SE Oak St., turn left onto SE 2nd Ave. to reach the imposing, mustard-yellow Olympic Mills Commerce Center, one of the more attractive structures in the area. Renovated and retrofitted in 2008, this large, open-format industrial space was originally the Olympic Cereal Mill, built in 1920. During the 1920s it was home to a General Mills subsidiary that churned out boxes of Wheaties. Today its tenants include, among other things, the highbrow charcuterie joint Olympic Provisions, which is about as far from a box of cereal as it's possible to get.

• Continue along SE 2nd Ave. and turn left at SE Morrison St. At the corner of Morrison and SE 3rd Ave. is Le Bistro Montage, whose mere name elicits gazes of dreamy nostalgia in Portland scenesters of a certain age. It was the ultimate late-night postclub dining spot during the 1990s (it opened in 1992 and was named Restaurant of the Year that year by local alt-weekly *Willamette Week*). It was, and still is, open for dinner until 4 a.m. Fridays and Saturdays, catering largely to the wasted and famished. Things that made it brilliant include white-clothed communal tables, "pounder" bottles of Rainier, frog legs, extremely cheap mac-and-cheese with odd enhancements such as Spam, oyster shooters (if you asked for one, the waiters would bellow your order to the kitchen at the tops of their lungs), *The Last Supper* and other humongous paintings on the walls, red wine in little jelly jars, and the swan and other animal-shaped tinfoil packages your leftovers would be wrapped in. (Most of which is still true, but fashions change; Montage no longer seems to be the place where *everyone* must appear after the bars close.)

- Turn right on SE 3rd Ave., then right again on SE Belmont St. to walk on the cobbled streets underneath the bridge ramp, between the columns. This part of town seems built for a Hollywood car chase. At SE Water Ave. turn left to pass the Hair of the Dog Brewing Company, home of one of Portland's first and still most highly regarded microbrewers. Stop in for a taste or a tour. Just ahead you'll see the Eastbank Commerce Center, another attractive and newish, or at least newly renovated, ware-house building. Across the street, its sibling, the Water Avenue Commerce Center, is home to the excellent Water Avenue Coffee. (The small roastery-café's alluring blue neon COFFEE sign beckons the undercaffeinated at all hours; the coffee can also be found in several Portland cafés and restaurants.)

- Turn left on SE Taylor St., then take a right on SE 2nd Ave.

- Follow SE 2nd through a few industrial blocks; at SE Clay St., take a right. When you get back to SE Water Ave., turn left and follow Water to the parking lot of the Oregon Museum of Science and Industry (OMSI).

- OMSI sits perched over the river at the southern end of the Eastside Industrial district. It's a great resource for anyone with kids, partly because, like a good Pixar movie, it's also fun for adults. The building, transformed from an old power plant, opened in 1992, but parts of the collection are much older, having belonged to the Portland Free Museum before being moved to OMSI at its old location near the zoo. These days, the museum hosts a number of permanent and rotating exhibitions, most of them with hands-on elements and all of them educational in a nonintimidating, science-is-fun kind of way (a regular installation on snot is a big early-winter draw). There's also a planetarium, an IMAX theater, and the submarine from *The Hunt for Red October*.

● To get back to your starting point, retrace your steps to SE Hawthorne Blvd., turn right, and catch MAX Light Rail at SE Grand Ave. Get off at E. Burnside St. and walk back up to NE 12th Ave.

POINTS OF INTEREST (START TO FINISH)

Hippo Hardware hippohardware.com, 1040 E. Burnside St., 503-231-1444

Jupiter Hotel jupiterhotel.com, 800 E. Burnside St., 503-230-9200

Doug Fir Lounge dougfirlounge.com, 830 E. Burnside St., 503-231-9663

Le Pigeon lepigeon.com, 738 E. Burnside St., 503-546-8796

Stark's Vacuum Museum starks.com, 107 NE Grand Ave., 800-230-4101

Burnside Skatepark East side of Burnside Bridge

Sheridan Fruit Company sheridanfruit.com, 409 SE Martin Luther King Jr. Blvd., 503-236-2114

Produce Row Café producerowcafe.com, 204 SE Oak St., 503-232-8355

Olympic Mills Commerce Center 107 SE Washington St.

Le Bistro Montage montageportland.com, 301 SE Morrison St., 503-234-1324

Hair of the Dog Brewing Company hairofthedog.com, 61 SE Water Ave., 503-232-6585

Water Avenue Coffee wateravenuecoffee.com, 1028 SE Water Ave., 503-808-7083

Oregon Museum of Science and Industry omsi.edu, 1945 SE Water Ave., 503-797-4640

ROUTE SUMMARY

1. Start at NE Couch St. and 12th Ave.
2. Turn left on NE 12th Ave. and cross E. Burnside St.
3. Turn right on E. Burnside.
4. Turn right on NE 6th Ave.
5. Turn left on NE Couch St.
6. Turn left on NE Martin Luther King Jr. Blvd.
7. Turn right on E. Burnside.

8. Retrace your steps up E. Burnside and turn right on SE 3rd Ave.

9. Turn left on SE Ankeny St.

10. Turn right on SE MLK Jr. Blvd.

11. Turn right on SE Oak St.

12. Turn left on SE 2nd Ave.

13. Turn left on SE Morrison St.

14. Turn right on SE 3rd Ave.

15. Turn right on SE Belmont St.

16. Turn left at SE Water Ave.

17. Turn left on SE Taylor St.

18. Turn right at SE 2nd Ave.

19. Turn right on SE Clay St.

20. Turn left on SE Water Ave. Route ends at OMSI.

CONNECTING THE WALKS

This walk links easily with Walk 10: Hawthorne Bridge to Steel Bridge, as well as with Walk 14: Hawthorne Blvd.

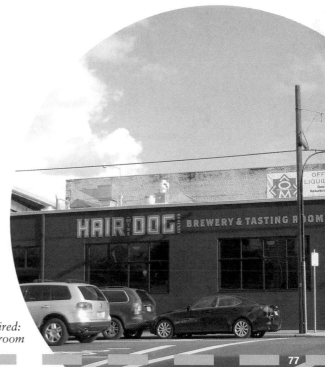

Hangover not required:
Hair of the Dog, a brewery and tasting room

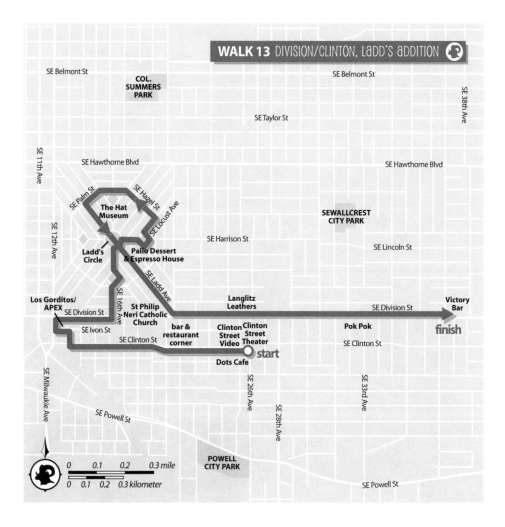

WALK 13 DIVISION/CLINTON, LADD'S ADDITION

SE Belmont St

COL. SUMMERS PARK

SE Belmont St

SE 38th Ave

SE Taylor St

SE 11th Ave

SE Hawthorne Blvd

SE Hawthorne Blvd

SE Palm St

SE Hazel St

The Hat Museum

SE Locust Ave

SEWALLCREST CITY PARK

SE 12th Ave

SE Harrison St

SE Lincoln St

Ladd's Circle

Pallo Dessert & Espresso House

SE Ladd Ave

Los Gorditos/ APEX

SE 16th Ave

Langlitz Leathers

SE Division St

Victory Bar

SE Division St

St Philip Neri Catholic Church

bar & restaurant corner

Clinton Street Video

Clinton Street Theater

Pok Pok

finish

SE Ivon St

SE Clinton St

SE Clinton St

Dots Cafe

start

SE Milwaukie Ave

SE 26th Ave

SE 28th Ave

SE 33rd Ave

SE Powell St

POWELL CITY PARK

SE Powell St

0   0.1   0.2   0.3 mile

0   0.1   0.2   0.3 kilometer

13 DIVISION/CLINTON, LaDD'S aDDITION: THeaTer of THe STreeT

BOUNDARIES: **SE 12th Ave., SE Hawthorne Blvd., SE 39th Ave., SE Clinton St.**
DISTANCE: **About 3.25 miles**
DIFFICULTY: **Easy**
PARKING: **Free street parking**
PUBLIC TRANSIT: **TriMet Bus 10 (SE Clinton St. and 26th Ave.) or Bus 4 (SE Division and 37th Ave.)**

A little pocket of Southeast Portland cool, the Division/Clinton area has been steadily gaining ground in recent years as a food-and-nightlife destination. Slick new apartment buildings have cropped up alongside bars and restaurants by the handful, in what just a few years ago was a cheap, mostly residential, totally unglamorous neighborhood. One result of all the activity is that already too-narrow Division Street has become a pedestrian-dodging gauntlet for drivers, and on-street parking is a hot enough commodity that local residents have lodged complaints against new apartment buildings being designed without parking spaces. But ultimately, of course, so much development and new business is good news for this area—if nothing else, it makes for a diverting walk with plenty of inviting places to linger and refuel. This walk also includes one of the city's prettiest residential areas, the labyrinthine Ladd's Addition, a small, historic neighborhood whose skewed angle and repeating pattern of diamond-shaped rose gardens make it almost as disorienting as it is attractive.

● Start at one of the early anchors of the tiny Clinton neighborhood, the Clinton Street Theater. Though it has changed hands frequently over the years, the Clinton has maintained a fairly consistent aesthetic sensibility, one that embraces the fringe of independent cinema. And we don't mean "fringe" and "independent" as in Sundance; we mean everything from Japanese gore-horror to local filmed-by-bike shorts to low-budget music documentaries. The theater's claim to fame, however—and its sustaining force—is *The Rocky Horror Picture Show,* which the Clinton has screened at midnight every Saturday since time began, more or less. If you've never seen *Rocky Horror,* it's worth investigating, if only for the vivid characters waiting in line to buy tickets.

- Across the street are two other great Portland institutions: Dots Cafe, a dimly lit, red-brocade-wallpapered restaurant-bar decorated with velvet matador paintings (it recently changed ownership but seems to be going strong and largely unchanged); and Clinton Street Video, one of the last independent video stores in town (or any-where, for that matter). It's owned by Chris Slusarenko, whose decades-deep roots in the local music scene—he fronted Sub Pop Records band Sprinkler in the early 1990s and played bass on the latest Guided By Voices tour—may help explain the store's killer inventory of all things music-related.

- From here, turn left to head west along SE Clinton St. At SE 21st Ave., you'll reach a little hub of lively bars and restaurants that have all cropped up in the past few years. A good choice for both food and drinks is the Night Light Lounge, one of the groundbreakers on this corner, with its romantic lighting, comfy couches in the back room, and mostly enclosed outdoor seating on the patio.

- Continue down SE Clinton St. to SE 13th Ave. and turn right. (Note the perfectly typi-cal Southeast Portland house on the corner as you turn.) At SE Ivon St. go left, then turn right on SE 12th Ave. At the end of the block on your right you'll come to the delightful eat–drink combo that is Los Gorditos taqueria and Apex bar. Round the corner to the right at SE Division St., then go on in and refresh yourself. The taqueria started as a popular food cart, still in its original location farther up Division, at SE 50th Ave. As for Apex, it has so many beers on tap that its computerized beer menu looks like the arrivals-and-departures board at an airport; it doesn't serve food, but you're allowed and encouraged to bring in edibles from Los Gorditos next door.

- Continue walking east up SE Division St. and hang a left at SE 16th Ave. to wander into the Ladd's Addition area. Notice on the right the St. Philip Neri Catholic Church complex, part of which was designed by architect Pietro Belluschi, whose fingerprints, you'll come to discover, are all over the city. (The original church was built by Joseph Jacobberger in 1913; Belluschi's addition is from 1949.)

- In two blocks you'll reach the first of the funky, slightly askew green spaces that make Ladd's Addition both wonderful and deeply confusing. It's easy to lose your way in this tangled nest of streets, but on the other hand, this is kind of a nice place in which to be lost. Ladd's Addition is Portland's oldest planned residential neighborhood; it has been a designated historic district with the National Register of Historic Places since 1988. It's roughly pinwheel-shaped, with four diamond-shaped green spaces and a central park area that all hold rose test gardens, and tree-lined residential streets in between, with homes built primarily from 1905 to 1930. The neighborhood is named after William Ladd, a merchant and mid-19th-century Portland mayor whose farm was here. (See Back Story: William S. Ladd, next page.)

- When you get to the first of the diamond-shaped green spaces, walk around it on the right-hand side and continue straight along SE 16th Ave. You'll soon reach Ladd's Circle, the main parklike hub. Turn right here; pass SE Ladd Ave., and note Palio Dessert & Espresso House on the right. One of the very few businesses within Ladd's Addition, Palio is open until 11 p.m., unusual for a coffee shop in Portland; the back room is lined with books, adding to the quiet, library-esque atmosphere of the place. Turn right on SE Harrison St., then right again on SE Cypress St.; then take two quick lefts to circumnavigate the rose-garden patch. You'll end up on SE Locust Ave.; turn right here, walk two blocks, then go left on SE Hazel St. Follow Hazel until it becomes the Holly St.–16th Ave. Alley.

The alleys in Ladd's Addition were initially planned as back-door service roads for the upper-crust homes envisioned here. (You'll walk right behind one such home between SE Poplar St. and 16th Ave.; it has the block to itself.) Today the alleys are considered public rights-of-way, open to foot and vehicle traffic, but most are unmaintained.

- Cross SE 16th Ave. and stay in the alley for another block; cross SE Maple St. to continue on SE Palm St. Turn left at SE Ladd Ave. On your left, in an unassuming bungalow, is the quirky Hat Museum (open by appointment only, $15 admission). Inside the 1910 Craftsman-style Ladd-Reingold House is a collection of not just hats but all sorts of random-seeming miscellany. Be prepared for eccentricity (and mermaids).

- Walk across Ladd's Circle and continue along elm-lined SE Ladd Ave. When you reach the three-way intersection of Ladd Ave., SE 20th Ave., and SE Division St., turn left to walk up Division.

- On the left, at SE Division and 25th Ave. (across from the legitimately divey Reel M Inn bar), you'll see Langlitz Leathers, one of Portland's coolest home-grown businesses. Ross Langlitz started it in 1947 after making his own protective gear for his

Back Story: William S. Ladd

It's not easy to imagine what Portland must've looked like when 24-year-old William Ladd arrived, in 1851, from New Hampshire with a shipment of booze to sell. But Ladd's impact on the way the city looks today is clear: he's at least partly responsible for some of its most beautiful areas, including Laurelhurst Park, Ladd's Addition, and the Crystal Springs Rhododendron Garden.

When Ladd made his way here, it was two years after gold had been found in California, and Portland was not much more than a rest area on the way to San Francisco, or a place where those who'd struck out could pause and lick their wounds. A census from around that time—December 1850— put the city's population at 821.

Ladd quickly made a name for himself. He set up shop immediately selling the liquor he'd brought, but within just a few days he had expanded his range of goods. Apparently he knew what he was doing. By 1853 he was able to build a storefront on Front Avenue, the first one made of brick in Portland. Teaming up with other investors, in the next several years he started railroad, shipping, manufacturing, and telegraph companies, not to mention the public library and River View Cemetery. With his original East Coast business partner, he founded the Ladd and Tilton Bank, Portland's first, in 1859. Ladd served as Portland's mayor from 1854 to 1855. He remained a well-regarded civic leader and businessman until he died.

Ladd was buried in River View Cemetery on January 9, 1893. In a bizarre coda, a few years later a caretaker found that his grave had been dug up and the body was missing. Ladd's remains, which had been taken for ransom, were eventually tracked down to the west side of the Willamette River, along what is now Macadam Avenue, and the thieves were arrested. He was reburied at River View—this time in cement.

motorcycle-racing habit (he was a devoted rider all his life, despite having lost a leg in a motorcycle accident at age 17). Langlitz jackets these days are internationally sought-after, but it's still a family business (Ross's granddaughter runs it now). Pop in and check out Ross's beloved Velocette hanging from the ceiling.

- Continue walking up SE Division St., through increasing numbers of new businesses, mostly bars and restaurants. This neighborhood has really picked up in recent years; it's officially a destination now, at least partly thanks to celebrated chef Andy Ricker's Thai restaurant Pok Pok, which has built an empire on a pile of chicken wings. Pok Pok started as a rickety little takeout shack in front of Ricker's house, with a brief menu inspired by some of the culinary revelations he had encountered as a young backpacker in the 1980s. The place quickly became so popular he had to expand it into the rest of the house. (He's since also opened a wildly beloved location in Brooklyn and one in Manhattan that specializes in pad Thai). You'll see Pok Pok on your right as you cross SE 32nd Ave. Diagonally across Division St. is its companion bar, the Whiskey Soda Lounge, which Ricker conceived as a place for "the drinking foods of Thailand"; it serves as a comfortable place to wait for a table at the restaurant. (You can get many of the Pok Pok dishes here, too.) Ricker is currently planning to open a curry house in this same area, a few blocks east.

- At the corner of SE Division St. and 37th Ave. is the Victory Bar, a nice stopping point, with an ace menu of comfort food (hush puppies, baked spaetzle) and bartenders with stellar cocktail-mixing pedigrees.

- From here you can take TriMet Bus 4 back down to SE Division and 26th Ave., then walk two blocks south to return to the starting point.

POINTS OF INTEREST (START TO FINISH)

Clinton Street Theater cstpdx.com, 2522 SE Clinton St., 503-238-5588

Dots Cafe 2521 SE Clinton St., 503-235-0203

Clinton Street Video 2501 SE Clinton St., 503-236-9030

Night Light Lounge nightlightlounge.net, 2100 SE Clinton St., 503-731-6500

Los Gorditos losgorditospdx.com, 1212 SE Division St., 503-445-6289

Apex apexbar.com, 1216 SE Division St., 503-273-9227

St. Philip Neri Catholic Church stphilipneripdx.org, 2408 SE 16th Ave., 503-231-4955

Palio Dessert & Espresso House palio-in-ladds.com, 1996 SE Ladd Ave., 503-232-9412

The Hat Museum thehatmuseum.com, 1928 SE Ladd Ave., 503-232-0433

Langlitz Leathers langlitz.com, 2443 SE Division St., 503-235-0959

Pok Pok pokpokpdx.com, 3226 SE Division St., 503-232-1387

Victory Bar thevictorybar.com, 3652 SE Division St., 503-236-8755

route summary

1. Start at the Clinton Street Theater, SE Clinton St. and 26th Ave.
2. Turn left on SE Clinton St., heading west.
3. Turn right on SE 13th Ave.
4. Turn left on SE Ivon St.
5. Turn right on SE 12th Ave.
6. Turn right on SE Division St.
7. Turn left on SE 16th Ave.
8. Turn right on Ladd's Circle.
9. Turn right on SE Harrison St.
10. Turn right on SE Cypress St.
11. Make two lefts to SE Locust Ave.
12. Turn right on SE Locust Ave.
13. Turn left on SE Hazel St.
14. Turn left on SE Ladd Ave.
15. Turn left on SE Division St.

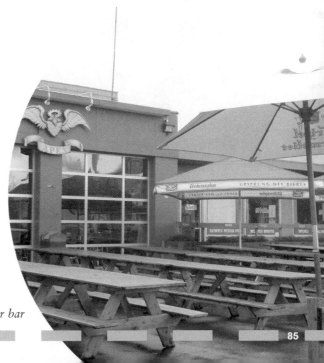

The patio of Apex beer bar

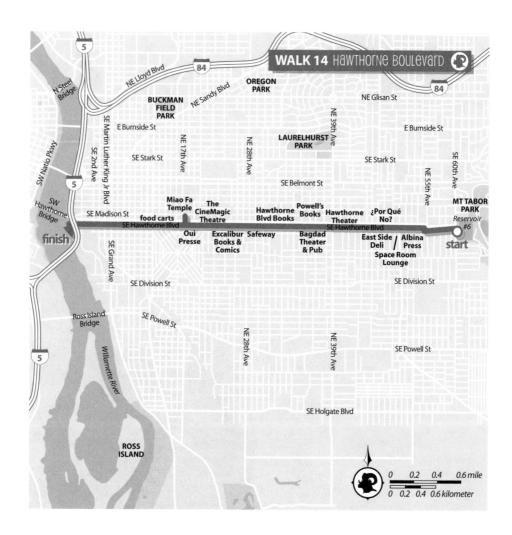

WALK 14 Hawthorne Boulevard

5

NE Lloyd Blvd

84

OREGON
PARK

NE Glisan St

N Steel
Bridge

NE Sandy Blvd

BUCKMAN
FIELD
PARK

SE Martin Luther King Jr Blvd

E Burnside St

NE 39th Ave

E Burnside St

SW Natio Pkwy

SE 2nd Ave

SE Stark St

NE 17th Ave

NE 28th Ave

LAURELHURST
PARK

SE Stark St

NE 55th Ave

SE 60th Ave

5

SE Belmont St

SW
Hawthorne
Bridge

SW

SE Madison St

Miao Fa
Temple

food carts

The
CineMagic
Theatre

Hawthorne
Blvd Books

Powell's
Books

Hawthorne
Theater

¿Por Qué
No?

MT TABOR
PARK

Reservoir
#6

SE Hawthorne Blvd

SE Hawthorne Blvd

finish

Oui
Presse

Excalibur
Books &
Comics

Safeway

Bagdad
Theater
& Pub

East Side
Deli

Albina
Press

start

SE Grand Ave

Space Room
Lounge

SE Division St

SE Division St

Ross Island
Bridge

SE Powell St

NE 28th Ave

NE 39th Ave

SE Powell St

Willamette River

5

SE Holgate Blvd

ROSS
ISLAND

0   0.2   0.4   0.6 mile

0   0.2 0.4 0.6 kilometer

14 HawTHOrNe BOULevard: Tabor To THe river

BOUNDARIES: SE Hawthorne Blvd., SE 60th Ave., Willamette River
DISTANCE: 3.5 miles
DIFFICULTY: Easy; moderate if done in reverse
PARKING: Free street parking
PUBLIC TRANSIT: TriMet Bus 71 (SE 60th Ave. and Hawthorne) and Bus 14 (all along Hawthorne)

When Portlanders talk about "Hawthorne," as in the district, they're usually thinking of a fairly small section of this major Southeast thoroughfare, from about 30th to 39th Avenues. In these few blocks you're likely to have to step gingerly over a few neo-hippies and their pets, feeling your way through clouds of patchouli and coming to terms with the idea of Caucasian dreadlocks. There are bead shops, burnouts, and occasional didjeridoos. Perhaps fittingly, the street and district are named for the founder of Oregon's first mental hospital (see Back Story: Dr. James C. Hawthorne on page 62); the street was once called Asylum Street. But there's much more to Hawthorne than its popular image. The street bisects Southeast Portland in all its multilayered glory, from the volcano to the river, from artistry to industry, as you'll quickly discover on this walk. (For more of a workout, try the route in reverse—it's on a slight but noticeable incline, and you can scamper to the top of Mt. Tabor if you haven't had enough by the time you reach the end.)

● Start at the stairs leading from SE 60th Ave. up the hill to Reservoir #6 on Mt. Tabor. If you're feeling sprightly, hop up the staircase for a view across town; if you're really energetic, take the *next* set of stairs as well for an even better view from a reservoir one level higher. Mt. Tabor is a dormant volcano, and the park that occupies it is one of the jewels of the city; it's a fantastic and very easily accessible bit of wilderness in which to stroll around, have a picnic, walk the dog, or get a workout. And the views from its higher reaches are spectacular in several directions. (Mt. Tabor is also the location of the annual Portland Adult Soapbox Derby—see Back Story on page 90.)

● Once back on SE 60th Ave., hang a right to reach SE Hawthorne Blvd., then turn left down Hawthorne. There's a little kink at SE 55th Ave.; veer right, then turn left again to stay on Hawthorne. (The small collection of buildings on your right at SE 56th Ave. make up the Portland campus of Western Seminary, an evangelical school.)

● At SE 50th Ave. you'll come to a couple of worthy stops, next door to each other on the left: Albina Press, where expert baristas churn out impeccable coffee in an open, gallery-like space (which in fact acts as a gallery, with art exhibitions that change once a month); and the Sapphire Hotel, a cozy, romantic wine bar with uncommonly attractive servers and a decadent opium-den feel. Both are excellent places to bring a date, if you're looking.

● Now leave all that sophistication behind you, because you'll have no use for it on the block between SE 48th and 49th Aves. This compact barhopping zone can do you serious damage if you're not careful: the establishments here are known (and sought out, especially by young 20-somethings and part-time pirates) for their liver-destroying qualities. Best to approach with caution. A good/terrible place to start is the Space Room Lounge; it's famous for hawking gigantic and needlessly robust Long Island iced tea in fishbowl glasses (if that tells you anything) and for the black-light murals of outer space that begin to look worryingly normal after a short time. Poke your head into a few of the other bars on the block, too, for future reference. (For an old-school unpretentious semipunk hangout, try Bar of the Gods, across the street.) And fear not: the next block holds several refueling options, including the rightly famous ¿Por Qué No? and the should-be-more-famous East Side Deli. Load up.

● Continue making your perhaps-now-crooked way along Hawthorne. Crossing SE 39th Ave., you'll see the Hawthorne Theatre building. These days it's a rock club, bar, and Chinese restaurant, but originally it was the Sunnyside Masonic Temple, built in 1919.

● A densely packed shopping (and dining) strip extends from SE 39th Ave. down to about 32nd; here you'll find everything from beads to vintage furniture and clothing to quirky gifts to American Apparel. Powell's Books (whose main location takes up a whole downtown city block) has a store here, on the right near SE 37th Ave., as well as an adjoining shop specializing in books for cooks and gardeners. And while we're talking books, mystery and crime-writing fans will want to take a moment of silence for Murder by the Book, down at 32nd Ave. This much-loved used-and-new-book store has sadly announced plans to close (though the owners were still hoping, at press time, to find a buyer) after several years of struggling to get by in a tough market. There's a chance it will have been rescued by the time you read this, but for now its future looks bleak.

- At SE 37th Ave. is a favorite Portland landmark, the Bagdad Theater & Pub, which more or less anchors this neighborhood. Built in 1927, partly funded by Universal Pictures, it's now owned by the local McMenamins chain and shows second-run movies in addition to hosting various events, readings, lectures, and more. The onion-topped neon sign is a good indication of the awesome Mediterranean-style interior; few movie palaces from this era retain their original glory, but this one does. (A plus: if you duck around the corner of the theater on 37th Ave., you'll find two more bars in the same building: the adorable and tiny cigar bar Greater Trumps and the big, boxy, echoey Backstage. Both are worth checking out.)

- Continue wandering down Hawthorne Blvd., investigating the various shops and restaurants as you see fit. Just past SE 32nd Ave. you'll come to Hawthorne Boulevard Books, a cute little used-book shop inside a small white house. On the next block is Hostelling International's Hawthorne Portland Hostel, a Hawthorne-ized bungalow from 1909 (dorm beds are $20–$24). The building has an ecoroof, a weird little clay-pagoda thing, and a stage in the huge backyard; it consistently wins sustainability awards, and it hosts a number of community-building events throughout the year (a bike-in movie night, travel-writing workshops, and the like). In contrast, a bit farther along, at SE 28th Ave., you'll come to a brand-new Safeway supermarket building that sticks out like a sore thumb in this bohemian neighborhood. The huge suburban fortress replaced a mid-1960s Safeway that had 20,000 fewer square feet and was certainly no beauty, but at least didn't impose itself on the surrounding blocks like an obnoxious beige-and-terra-cotta bully.

Taking in the view at Mt. Tabor Park
(Photo courtesy of Paul Gerald)

Back Story: Portland Adult Soapbox Derby

Held on the slopes of Mt. Tabor, usually on a Saturday in mid-August, the Portland Adult Soapbox Derby is a favorite local tradition. The derby in its current incarnation started in 1997, inspired by a visit to San Francisco's annual Bernal Heights version. These days, thousands of spectators line the race course, brandishing tall cans of watery domestic beer as they loudly egg on the teams of racers. Forty-odd teams participate, building cars designed either for speed or for show (sometimes both). Themed cars have included a miniature Sandy Hut, complete with bartender; a fully lit stage with a band on it, performing all the way down the course; a tank; a rib cage; a kiddie pool; a big black Caddy; a taqueria serving tequila shots; a basketball court; a hot dog; and frequent winner Specific Gravity, which looks like a beautifully varnished handmade wooden canoe. The cars are powered by gravity only, and there's a limit to how much you can spend to build them (as well as rules about number of axles, type of wheels, allowable missiles, and so forth). Injuries are numerous and sometimes gruesome—epic road rash from being dragged down half the course beneath a car; a piece of flying metal to the face of a volunteer—but no one really complains. The derby's spirit is indomitable. The race usually lasts several hours, then culminates in a huge party somewhere near the foot of Mt. Tabor. It's free to watch. If you're in town when it's on, don't miss it. For details, visit **soapboxracer.com.**

● Moving quickly on, walk down the hill past the Holman Funeral Service building (from 1901 and very nice-looking) to reach Excalibur Books & Comics, one of the city's best comic-book shops. A few blocks down, at SE 23rd Ave., is Grand Central Bakery, with a handful of locations around town and in Seattle; its rustic Como bread debuted in the late 1980s and basically educated Pacific Northwesterners about artisanal baking.

- At SE 20th Ave. is yet another classic movie house, The CineMagic, a single-screen theater that opened in 1914. It's famous today for its teeny, adorable 1950s bathrooms and the awesome gold-lamé stage curtain (and, to some of us, for showing *The Secret of Roan Inish* for what seemed like decades but was really only about a year).

- Continue down Hawthorne. On the left at 18th Ave. you'll see Oui Presse, an impeccably curated magazine store, gift shop, bakery, and coffee/tea/wine bar next door to the highly regarded restaurant Castagna. Ask about the bunny slippers!

- Take a right onto SE 17th Ave. for one block. At SE 17th and Madison St. is the Miao Fa Temple, designed in 1926 by architect William Gray Purcell, who—not too surprisingly when you look at the building—once worked with Louis Sullivan, as well as other prominent Chicago architects. The building was originally a church but became a Buddhist temple in 1996. The more recently added Eastern-style embellishments (like bamboo roofing and the concrete lions guarding the entrance), juxtaposed with the clean-lined cube of the original building, make for a slightly trippy but somehow very pleasing sight.

- At the corner of SE 12th Ave. and Hawthorne is one of the original trendsetting food-cart "pods" that have made Portland a destination for street food. Mainstays here include the great Potato Champion (in a word, poutine; in several words, late-night postbar poutine) and Whiffies, a fried-pie cart.

- From here, it's a straight shot through lower, industrial Hawthorne to reach the Eastbank Esplanade. To get there, cross SE Grand Ave. and walk up onto the Hawthorne Bridge ramp as if you were going to cross the bridge. Just before the river, take the stairs leading down from the bridge onto the esplanade. (You could also simply walk toward the river at street level, underneath the bridge, but it's more fun to take the high road.)

- To return to the starting point, retrace your steps across SE Grand Ave. and hop onto TriMet Bus 14, at SE Hawthorne Blvd. and 6th Ave.

POINTS OF INTEREST (START TO FINISH)

Albina Press 5012 SE Hawthorne Blvd., 503-282-5214

Sapphire Hotel thesapphirehotel.com, 5008 SE Hawthorne Blvd., 503-232-6333

Space Room Lounge spaceroomlounge.com, 4800 SE Hawthorne Blvd., 503-235-6957

Bar of the Gods barofthegods.com, 4801 SE Hawthorne Blvd., 503-232-2037

¿Por Qué No? porquenotacos.com, 4635 SE Hawthorne Blvd., 503-954-3138

East Side Deli pdxdeli.com, 4626 SE Hawthorne Blvd., 503-236-7313

Hawthorne Theatre hawthornetheatre.com, 1507 SE 39th Ave., 503-233-7100

Powell's Books on Hawthorne powells.com, 3723 SE Hawthorne Blvd., 503-228-4651

Bagdad Theater & Pub mcmenamins.com/bagdad, 3702 SE Hawthorne Blvd., 503-467-7521

Murder by the Book mbtb.com, 3210 SE Hawthorne Blvd., 503-232-9995

Hawthorne Boulevard Books 3129 SE Hawthorne Blvd., 503-236-3211

Hawthorne Portland Hostel portlandhostel.org, 3031 SE Hawthorne Blvd., 503-236-3380

Excalibur Books & Comics excaliburcomics.net, 2444 SE Hawthorne Blvd., 503-231-7351

Grand Central Bakery grandcentralbakery.com, 2230 SE Hawthorne Blvd., 503-445-1600

The CineMagic Theatre thecinemagictheater.com, 2021 SE Hawthorne Blvd., 503-231-7919

Oui Presse oui-presse.com, 1740 SE Hawthorne Blvd., 503-384-2160

Castagna castagnarestaurant.com, 1752 SE Hawthorne Blvd., 503-231-7373

Miao Fa Temple miaofatemple.com, 1722 SE Madison St., 503-239-5678

route summary

1. Start near the corner of SE 60th and Hawthorne Blvd., at the stairs leading into Mt. Tabor Park.

2. Turn right (north) on SE 60th Ave.

3. Turn left on SE Hawthorne Blvd.

4. Turn right on SE 55th Ave.

5. Turn left on SE Hawthorne.

6. Cross SE Grand Ave. and walk onto the Hawthorne Bridge ramp.

7. Just before the river, take the stairs down from the bridge onto the Eastbank Esplanade.

connecting the walks

Follow SE 60th Ave. to join up with Walk 15: Stark-Belmont. Hop off Hawthorne at SE Grand Ave. to join the Walk 12: Industrial Southeast. At the Eastbank Esplanade, join Walk 10: Hawthorne Bridge to Steel Bridge.

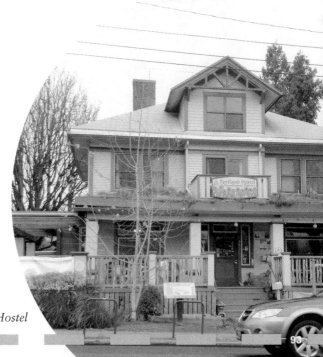

The eco-friendly Hawthorne Portland Hostel

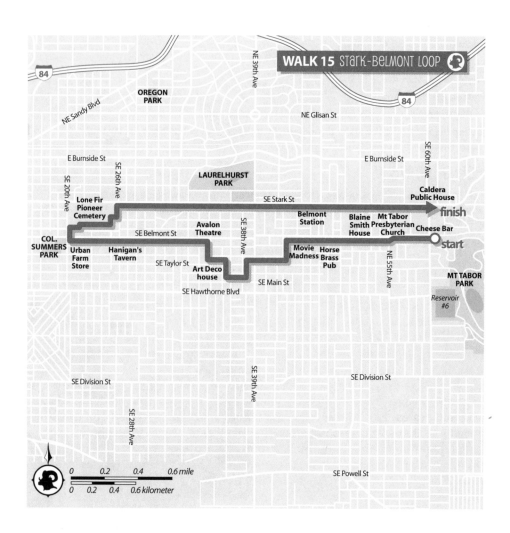

WALK 15 STARK-BELMONT LOOP

84

NE 39th Ave

OREGON
PARK

NE Sandy Blvd

NE Glisan St

84

E Burnside St

SE 26th Ave

E Burnside St

SE 60th Ave

LAURELHURST
PARK

Caldera
Public House

SE 20th Ave

Lone Fir
Pioneer
Cemetery

SE Stark St

finish

COL.
SUMMERS
PARK

SE Belmont St

Avalon
Theatre

SE 38th Ave

Belmont
Station

Blaine
Smith
House

Mt Tabor
Presbyterian
Church

Cheese Bar

start

Urban
Farm
Store

Hanigan's
Tavern

SE Taylor St

Art Deco
house

Movie
Madness

Horse
Brass
Pub

NE 55th Ave

MT TABOR
PARK

SE Hawthorne Blvd

SE Main St

Reservoir
#6

SE Division St

SE 28th Ave

SE 39th Ave

SE Division St

0   0.2   0.4   0.6 mile

0   0.2   0.4   0.6 kilometer

SE Powell St

15 Stark-Belmont: Heart of the Southeast

BOUNDARIES: **SE 60th Ave., SE Stark St., SE Belmont St., SE 20th Ave.**
DISTANCE: **5 miles**
DIFFICULTY: **Easy (moderate if you include Mt. Tabor)**
PARKING: **Free street parking**
PUBLIC TRANSIT: **TriMet Bus 15 runs along SE Belmont St. to/from downtown**

Where do ordinary, average Portlanders hang out? Well, there's really no such thing as a typical Portlander, despite what a certain TV sketch-comedy series might have you believe, but this walk takes in a couple of the residential neighborhoods that have a very Southeast Portland feel: moderate-size bungalows, nicely maintained yards with the occasional urban veggie farm or chicken coop, quiet tree-lined streets, chillaxed bars and restaurants where you can show up in jeans and not be looked at sideways. The houses are more modest as the street numbers get smaller (not counting one particularly ostentatious home we'll pause to gawk at). This is a nice walk to do in late afternoon or early evening, when it's not quite dark but the street life on Belmont is starting to pick up.

● **Start your walk at the corner of SE Belmont St. and 60th Ave., home of the Cheese Bar, a deli and specialty-cheese shop with an impressive beer and wine list. Up the hill is Mt. Tabor Park—if you have plenty of time, you might consider a picnic before you set out. Mt. Tabor, aside from being a wonderful place for a short hike, a picnic, walking your dog, training for cyclocross, or just lounging with a paperback, also happens to be an extinct volcano, part of the Boring Lava Field. (We're not judging—that's what it's called.) The park includes about 190 acres atop the cinder cone, covered with leafy trees, ferns, reservoirs, and a network of trails (paved and unpaved), plus a well-maintained playground area. The many sets of stairs leading up to its top are popular with runners and masochists. The park is also the location of the annual Portland Adult Soapbox Derby (see Back Story on page 90). Fun fact: the hill is named after a Mt. Tabor in Israel. Near the relatively flat top is a statue of Harvey Scott, who edited *The Oregonian* newspaper for several years starting in 1865. The statue was created by Danish-American sculptor Gutzon Borglum, whose credits include Mt. Rushmore. And in case you're the nervous type, fear not: the volcano hasn't been active for around 300,000 years, so you *should* be safe.**

- From the Cheese Bar, head west—downhill—along SE Belmont St. Where the road bends at SE 55th Ave., you'll see Mt. Tabor Presbyterian Church, whose hundred-year-old bell tower is now TaborSpace, a nonprofit, pay-what-you-like coffee shop and community center. The big Arts and Crafts–style mansion on the right as you continue down the hill is the Blaine Smith House (5219 SE Belmont), built in 1909 and listed on the National Register of Historic Places. Note how the houses and yards become gradually less majestic as you make your way down the hill.

- On your left, a few blocks farther down, is one of Portland's greatest drinking establishments, the Horse Brass Pub. Pop in for a Scotch egg and one of the gazillion excellent beers on tap. The rough-hewn wooden tables and smoke-patina'd walls give the place a convincing Old World feel.

- On the next block, just past the excellent Bicycle Repair Collective (which opened in 1976 and helped launch the city's radical-cyclist community) and a brand-new, teeny-tiny hat shop, is the city's coolest video store, Movie Madness, which doubles as a museum of film props and costumes. (Just how wide was Orson Welles in A *Touch of Evil*? Take a look at his jacket on display here, and you'll have a pretty good idea. For fun, compare it to Erich von Stroheim's getup from *Sunset Boulevard,* or an itty-bitty outfit worn by Natalie Wood.) Across the parking lot is one of Portland's countless "pods" of food carts, where you can get anything from gyros to waffles to beer and cappuccino—even, as of this writing, a Norwegian *lefse*-meatball wrap.

- At SE 42nd Ave., hang a left, walk two blocks to SE Taylor St., and turn right. Cross busy SE 39th Ave., renamed Cesar E. Chavez Blvd. in 2009 (after a surprisingly long and contentious debate), and at SE 38th Ave. duck through a little alley to the left. Take a right at SE Main St.

- At the corner of SE Main and 36th Ave. is an uncharacteristically ostentatious house worth a peek. A pale yellow Art Deco confection, it was built in 1992 by Paul Wenner, the man who invented the Gardenburger. (See Back Story: Gardenburger on page 98.)

- Take a right onto SE 36th Ave., a left on SE Taylor St., and a right on SE 35th Ave. to get back onto SE Belmont St., heading left (west). From about 35th to 33rd Aves.,

Belmont coalesces into a lively, fun-filled hub of bars, coffee shops, and a nickel arcade with a cheap-movie theater attached (the Avalon, whose neon sign you can't miss). There's an artisan-cupcake shop; a record store that's also a fussy cocktail lounge; a vegan bar in a former never-open mattress shop that everyone thought was a front for something shady; a place named after Finnish designer Alvar Aalto; and pizza. Explore!

● Continue along SE Belmont St. On your left, at SE 27th Ave., note Hanigan's Tavern, which has long been affectionately and unofficially known as "The Vern" because most of the letters in its sign burned out ages ago; it's also one of the very cheapest drinkeries in town. At 2100 SE Belmont you'll see the Urban Farm Store, another little slice of Portlandia. You haven't really made it in this town until you've installed a pair of chickens in your backyard.

● At SE 20th Ave. you'll be facing Col. Summers Park, which in summer becomes a horrorscape of pasty-skinned Portlanders exposing discon- certingly generous amounts of their Pabst-fueled bod- ies while playing Frisbee or Hacky Sack (yes, still, in 2013). There's also a big patch of community gardens here. The park, established in 1938, is named after Col. Owen Summers, an Oregon legislator known for having commanded the Second Oregon Volunteers Regiment during the Spanish-American War.

● Hang a right on SE 20th Ave. and cross SE Morrison St.; go right on Morrison, then, in half a block or so, duck left through the gate into Lone Fir Pioneer Cemetery. Founded in 1855, the cemetery started out as a farm; when the owner sold the land, his father was already buried here. Then a boiler explosion on a steamship belonging to the new

The Avalon Theatre, a second-run-movie house and mini-arcade on SE Belmont Street

Back Story: Gardenburger

Given Portland's image in the popular imagination, it's probably not a *huge* surprise that the Gardenburger was invented here. (Well, strictly speaking, it happened in Gresham, but let's not quibble.) The meatless patty is the brainchild of Paul Wenner, who (after becoming concerned about what his lousy diet was doing to his mood, energy levels, and physical well-being) opened a vegetarian restaurant in 1981 called The Gardenhouse. Looking for something to do with all the leftovers one night, he made a probably not enormous intuitive leap and came up with the "Gardenloaf Sandwich." A little more fine-tuning (slice and fry, basically) converted the loafwich into an early version of the Gardenburger.

Customers at the Gardenhouse seemed to love it—alas, the restaurant itself was not long for this world. Wenner closed up shop in the midst of a recession in 1984, but he was by no means out of the Gardenburger game. With financial backing from Harry Merlo, then CEO of Louisiana-Pacific,

Wenner started Wholesome & Hearty Foods Inc. and continued to produce his trademark veggie burger.

The company changed its name to Gardenburger Inc. in 1985; it grew quickly and went public in 1992. Throughout the 1990s, competition from Boca Burgers, MorningStar Farms, and other companies following in Gardenburger's footsteps started picking up. Feeling the pressure, Gardenburger spent about $1.5 million on an advertising spot on the final episode of *Seinfeld*. Even so, the company continued losing money over the next few years: its stock prices dropped from $18 to 50 cents a share, and finally, in 2005, Gardenburger declared bankruptcy. Kellogg purchased the brand in 2007 and still owns it.

As for Wenner, he's written a couple of healthy-eating cookbooks and is now marketing his latest invention, the Gardenbar—a protein snack bar that tastes like vegetables instead of dessert.

owner, Colburn Barrell, killed several people, including Barrell's business partner, and he buried them all near the original tenant, starting what he called Mount Crawford Cemetery. In 1866 Barrell sold the land to a group of investors, and it was renamed

Lone Fir for the one tree growing on the land. Now there are 25,000 people buried there, and a lot more than one tree. Like many urban cemeteries, it's a lovely, cool, quiet place to wander through. The area is fenced in, so aim diagonally for the gate at SE 26th Ave., on the east side.

● Exiting the cemetery, take a left at SE 26th Ave., then a right at SE Stark St. At Stark and SE 28th Ave., you can link with Walk 17: Kerns and Laurelhurst Park, or you can continue up Stark, bordering Laurelhurst Park, along a quiet, tree-lined residential street.

● Beer nerds should note Belmont Station, at SE Stark St. and 45th Ave., a bottle shop with a tiny pub attached. It's run by the same folks who operate the Horse Brass Pub. The variety of beer and hard cider available for purchase is astounding, and the shop also sells imported British snacks, in case you're fresh out of Twiglets or Marmite.

● The walk ends at Caldera Public House, a friendly brewpub serving upscale food and fine craft beers in the 1910 Thomas Graham building. (It was once a pharmacy and is now a historic landmark, and once upon a time it faced a streetcar line that ran up and down the hill.) Ignore the awful gray-and-taupe neo-blah multiuse building across the street.

● From Caldera, simply walk south on SE 60th Ave. to return to SE Belmont St. and our starting point.

POINTS OF INTEREST (START TO FINISH)

Cheese Bar cheese-bar.com, 6031 SE Belmont St., 503-222-6014 (closed Mondays)

TaborSpace taborspace.org, 5441 SE Belmont St., 503-238-3904

Horse Brass Pub horsebrass.com, 4534 SE Belmont St., 503-232-2202

Movie Madness moviemadnessvideo.com, 4320 SE Belmont St., 503-234-4363

Avalon Theatre and Wunderland wunderlandgames.com/avalontheatre.asp, 3451 SE Belmont St., 503-238-1617

Hanigan's Tavern (a.k.a. The Vern) 2622 SE Belmont St., 503-233-7851

BACK STORY: PIONEER CEMETERIES

Scattered about Portland are 14 historic pioneer cemeteries, which Metro maintains along with burial records for each of them. (The records have recently been digitized, and Metro allows people researching genealogy or family history to search them.) Many of the pioneer cemeteries are still active, though Lone Fir and a few others have been closed to new burials because all the spots are either taken or already owned.

Lone Fir is the oldest and largest of these cemeteries. Its "residents" include Thomas J. Dryer, the politician and mountain climber who founded the *Weekly Oregonian* newspaper; Asa Lovejoy, the founder of Portland, who lost the coin toss—he'd have named it Boston; Esther Lovejoy, suffragette and physician; and Georgiana Pittock, of Pittock Mansion fame.

Most of the cemeteries were established between 1850 and 1870, when California gold fever and the promise of land up for grabs drew the desperate and/or brave from the East Coast toward the Oregon Territory. As one might imagine, this was no easy trip; many of those who set out did not make it, and many others didn't last long once they got here. The cemeteries today make for beautifully quiet, peaceful, atmospheric escapes from the city. For details, visit Metro's website on the topic: **tinyurl.com /pdxpioneercemeteries.**

Urban Farm Store urbanfarmstore.com, 2100 SE Belmont St., 503-234-7733

Lone Fir Pioneer Cemetery friendsoflonefircemetery.org, SE 26th Ave. between Stark and Morrison Sts.

Belmont Station belmont-station.com, 4500 SE Stark St., 503-232-8538

Caldera Public House calderapublichouse.com, 6031 SE Stark St., 503-233-8242

route summary

1. Start at the corner of SE 60th Ave. and Belmont St.
2. Head west along SE Belmont St.
3. Turn left on SE 42nd Ave.
4. Turn right on SE Taylor St.
5. Turn left through the alley at SE 38th Ave.
6. Turn right on SE Main St.
7. Turn right on SE 36th Ave.
8. Turn left on SE Taylor St.
9. Turn right on SE 35th Ave.
10. Turn left on SE Belmont St.
11. Turn right on SE 20th Ave.
12. Turn right on SE Morrison St.
13. Turn left into Lone Fir Pioneer Cemetery.
14. Turn left on SE 26th Ave.
15. Turn right on SE Stark St.
16. Follow SE Stark St. to SE 60th Ave.

connecting the walks

At SE 28th Ave. and Stark St., you can link with Walk 17: Kerns and Laurelhurst Park.

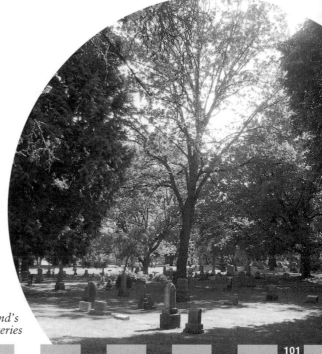

Lone Fir, the largest and oldest of Portland's pioneer cemeteries

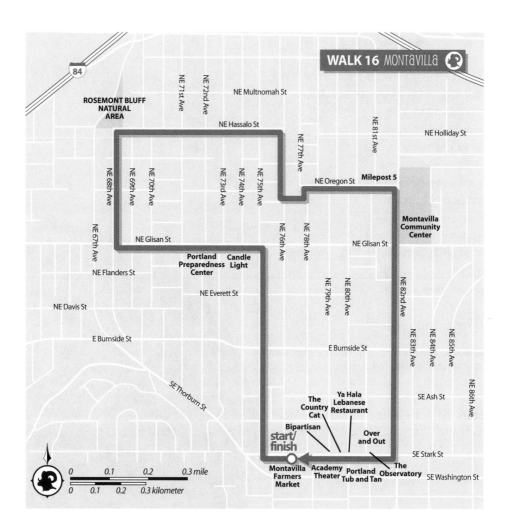

84

ROSEMONT BLUFF
NATURAL
AREA

NE 71st Ave

NE 72nd Ave

NE Multnomah St

NE Hassalo St

NE 68th Ave

NE 69th Ave

NE 70th Ave

NE 73rd Ave

NE 74th Ave

NE 75th Ave

NE 77th Ave

NE 81st Ave

NE Holliday St

NE Oregon St   Milepost 5

NE 67th Ave

NE Glisan St

NE 76th Ave

NE 78th Ave

Montavilla
Community
Center

NE Glisan St

Portland
Preparedness
Center

Candle
Light

NE Flanders St

NE Everett St

NE 79th Ave

NE 80th Ave

NE 82nd Ave

NE Davis St

E Burnside St

SE Thorburn St

E Burnside St

NE 83th Ave

NE 84th Ave

NE 85th Ave

NE 86th Ave

SE Ash St

Ya Hala
Lebanese
Restaurant

The
Country
Cat

Bipartisan

Over
and Out

SE Stark St

start/
finish

Montavilla
Farmers
Market

Academy
Theater

Portland
Tub and Tan

The
Observatory

SE Washington St

0   0.1   0.2   0.3 mile

0   0.1   0.2   0.3 kilometer

16 MONTAVILLA: a Stark Story

BOUNDARIES: **NE Hassalo St., 82nd Ave., SE Stark St., 75th Ave., NE Glisan St., NE 68th Ave.**
DISTANCE: **3 miles**
DIFFICULTY: **Easy**
PARKING: **Free street parking**
PUBLIC TRANSIT: **TriMet Bus 15 (SE Stark St. and 80th Ave., SE Washington St. and 76th Ave.)**

This up-and-coming little neighborhood, whose name is short for "Mt. Tabor Villa," has come a long way in recent years. Not too long ago it was at best neglected, at worst avoided, or even considered a little dodgy. As recently as 2008, neighborhood complaints about prostitution problems in the neighborhood—primarily along 82nd Avenue—led the city to form a volunteer advisory committee of concerned citizens to look into eliminating the problem. Prostitution hasn't gone away, but things generally have been improving for Montavilla, at least in the neighborhood's main commercial core, along Stark Street from 76th Avenue to 82nd Avenue or so. The farmers' market here is a big draw for locals as well as folks in other neighborhoods, as are several of the bars and restaurants that have opened up along here, not to mention the movie theater. Local residents have been lobbying for the past couple of years to establish a co-op grocery store in the area, not just for shopping but as an informal neighborhood community center where people could gather and meet each other; a volunteer organization called the Montavilla Food Co-Op is working toward raising funds and gathering info to make the community-owned grocery store idea a reality here. Meanwhile, the whole area is just minutes from the top of Mt. Tabor, an ideal playground and one of the city's best parks.

● Start the walk at the site of the Montavilla Farmers Market, at the corner of SE 76th Ave. and Stark St. (note that it's only open Sundays, 10 a.m.–2 p.m., June–October, plus a handful of dates throughout the winter months). Head west on SE Stark St. to 75th Ave. and turn right. Follow 75th for several blocks until you reach Glisan St., where you'll turn left. This little stretch of Glisan has a few appealing places to stop for refueling, including the old-school diner-lounge combo that is the Candlelight (recommended mostly for drinks and supercheap dive-bar breakfasts, FYI). But most of the businesses along here are strictly utilitarian: do your taxes, fix your car, get ready for the coming apocalypse. That last would be a reference to the somewhat mystifying Portland Preparedness Center, a business dedicated to making sure we all have what we need when the zombies attack/the aliens arrive/the earthquake destroys the city. Better safe than sorry!

- At NE 68th Ave., turn right for several blocks. At the corner of NE 68th and Hassalo St. you'll come to the 2-acre Rosemont Bluff Natural Area, a sort of buffer zone of undeveloped woodland and wildlife habitat covering a steep slope. It's naturally populated with Douglas-fir and maple, but invasive ivy and blackberry plants are a constant problem, so neighbors volunteer frequently to help maintain the park. (This neighborhood is technically not part of Montavilla but rather North Tabor or Center; "Center" started out as an acronym that stood for "Citizens Engaged Now Towards Ecological Review.")

- Turn right on NE Hassalo St. At NE 76th Ave., turn right again. Turn left on NE Irving St.; walk a block, then turn left again on NE 78th Ave., and then turn right on NE Oregon St. Where Oregon meets NE 82nd Ave., you'll come to Milepost 5, a cool multi-use space that incorporates live–work art studios and galleries. Stroll the complex, taking in the artwork, or check the website for a calendar of performances and events being held in the theater space.

- Turn right on NE 82nd Ave., one of the least glamorous streets in Portland—all fast-food restaurants, gas stations, and cheap motels. At the corner of NE Glisan St. is one welcome exception: the Montavilla Community Center. It has two outdoor pools, a basketball court, meeting rooms, classrooms, and a varied program of activities for both kids and adults.

- Continue along 82nd Ave., taking care not to make eye contact with passing cars lest they mistake you for someone selling one or another category of illicit goods and services. Just as you begin to suspect that you're trudging headlong into Portland's used-car-sales territory, you'll come to SE Stark St. Turn right onto Stark. There's a semisecret neighborhood bar nearby; to find it, traverse the McDonald's parking lot and walk around to the back of the building next door, until you come to a glass door. This is the Over and Out, the back bar hidden behind an upscale restaurant and cocktail bar called The Observatory. (You could also go in the front door, on Stark St., and walk through the restaurant to the back, but that's somehow less exciting.) The

Over and Out is a boxy, relaxed space with pool tables and pinball, an excellent cocktail menu, and several of the same food items you can get in the restaurant (plus a great happy-hour selection).

- Continue to make your way along SE Stark St., which as you'll notice is a small but recently expanding commercial stretch, with fancy new cocktail lounges and bike shops mixed in among places that have been here since before it was cool, like Portland Tub and Tan. (Hot tubs by the hour? Nothing sketchy about that whatsoever!) On the right, just before SE 80th Ave., is Ya Hala Lebanese Restaurant, an excellent choice if you're hungry; it's one of the longer-established restaurants along this stretch. Next door to it, and owned by the same friendly family, is a small international grocery and supplies store, where you can get orange-flower water, gorgeous-smelling olive soap, Mediterranean cooking supplies, cheese, tea and spices, baked goods, and many other things.

- In the next block of Stark is The Country Cat, one of the first restaurants here to get attention from folks outside the neighborhood. The family-owned place serves snazzed-up home-style American classics for dinner nightly, but it's perhaps even more universally loved as a brunch spot. At the end of the block is the Bipartisan Cafe, a stellar coffee shop that also makes fantastic pies and pastries. Like pretty much all of the businesses on this stretch, both of these places are noticeably kid-friendly; The Country Cat has a children's menu, and the Bipartisan has a play corner and is usually full of at least as many strollers as laptops.

- Diagonally across the street from the Bipartisan is another of Portland's great beer-and-pizza second-run movie houses, the Academy Theater. Built originally in 1948 as a single-screen theater, it had been closed and languishing since the 1970s before it was bought, restored, and reopened in 2006 as a multiscreen second-run theater and pub. (Along with 10 microbrews on tap, the theater serves pizza from the next-door Flying Pie Pizzeria, an old-school favorite.) It's both kid- and parent-friendly: before 8 p.m. the theater offers babysitting services, which means you only have to watch that Disney-princess movie if you *really* want to.

- Walk another block or so along SE Stark St. to return to the farmers' market and the route's starting point.

POINTS OF INTEREST (START TO FINISH)

Montavilla Farmers Market montavillamarket.org, 7600 block of SE Stark St.

Candlelight Restaurant & Lounge 7334 NE Glisan St., 503-253-9738

Portland Preparedness Center getreadyportland.com, 7202 NE Glisan St., 503-252-2525

Milepost 5 milepost5.net, 850 NE 81st Ave.

Montavilla Community Center 8219 NE Glisan St., 503-823-4101

Over and Out/The Observatory theobservatorypdx.com, 410 SE 81st Ave., 503-445-6284

Portland Tub and Tan tubandtan.com, 8028 SE Stark St., 503-261-1180

Ya Hala Lebanese Restaurant yahalarestaurant.com, 8005 SE Stark St., 503-256-4484

The Country Cat thecountrycat.net, 7937 SE Stark St., 503-408-1414

Bipartisan Cafe bipartisancafe.com, 7901 SE Stark St., 503-253-1051

Academy Theater academytheaterpdx.com, 7818 SE Stark St., 503-252-0500

Flying Pie Pizzeria flying-pie.com, 7804 SE Stark St., 503-254-2016

ROUTE SUMMARY

1. Start at the corner of SE 76th Ave. and Stark St.
2. Walk west on SE Stark.
3. Turn right at SE 75th Ave.
4. Turn left at NE Glisan St.
5. Turn right at NE 68th Ave.
6. Turn right at NE Hassalo St.
7. Turn right at NE 76th Ave.
8. Turn left at NE Irving St.
9. Turn left at NE 78th Ave.
10. Turn right at NE Oregon St.
11. Turn right at NE 82nd Ave.
12. Turn right at SE Stark St.

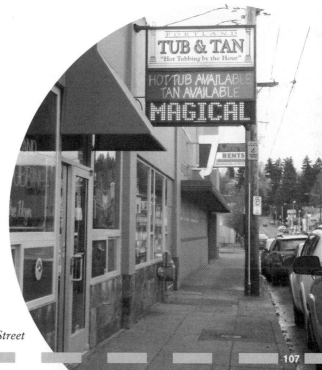

Portland Tub and Tan, on SE Stark Street

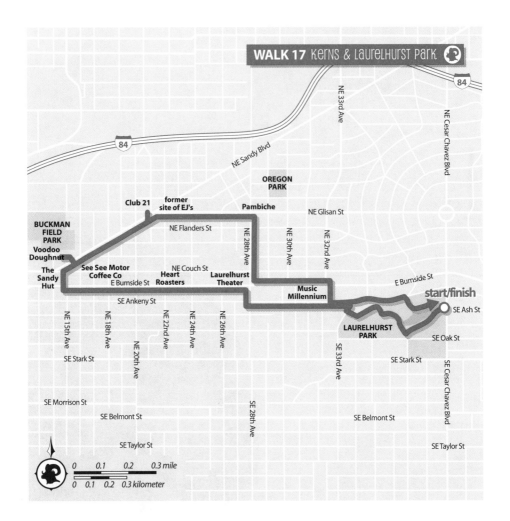

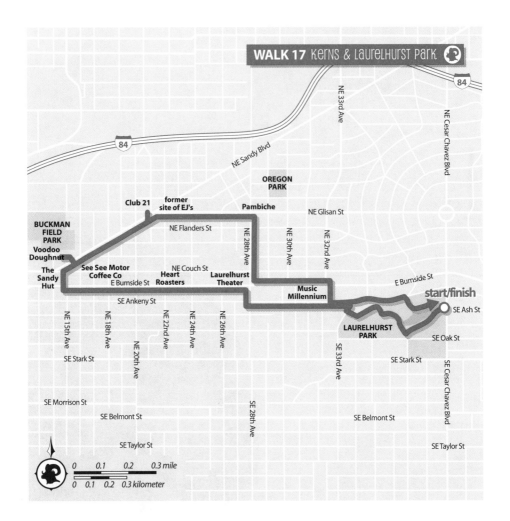WALK 17 Kerns & Laurelhurst Park

84

NE 33rd Ave

NE Cesar Chavez Blvd

84

NE Sandy Blvd

OREGON
PARK

Club 21　former
site of EJ's　Pambiche

NE Glisan St

NE 32nd Ave

BUCKMAN
FIELD
PARK

NE Flanders St

NE 30th Ave

Voodoo
Doughnut

NE 28th Ave

The
Sandy
Hut

See See Motor
Coffee Co

NE Couch St

E Burnside St

Heart
Roasters

Laurelhurst
Theater

E Burnside St

SE Ankeny St

Music
Millennium

start/finish

SE Ash St

NE 15th Ave

NE 18th Ave

NE 20th Ave

NE 22nd Ave

NE 24th Ave

NE 26th Ave

LAURELHURST
PARK

SE Oak St

SE Stark St

SE Stark St

NE 33rd Ave

SE Cesar Chavez Blvd

SE Morrison St

SE Belmont St

SE 28th Ave

SE Belmont St

SE Taylor St

SE Taylor St

0   0.1   0.2   0.3 mile
0   0.1   0.2   0.3 kilometer

17 Kerns and Laurelhurst Park: The Bermuda Triangle

BOUNDARIES: **SE Cesar Chavez Blvd., SE Stark St., NE 15th Ave., NE Sandy Blvd.**
DISTANCE: **3.5 miles**
DIFFICULTY: **Easy**
PARKING: **Free street parking**
PUBLIC TRANSIT: **TriMet Bus 75 (SE Cesar Chavez Blvd. and Ash St.)**

There are enough entertaining diversions on this walk that you may well never return from it. The route starts and stops at one of Portland's finest green spaces, the beautifully landscaped Laurelhurst Park. Surrounding the park are block after block of sturdy, dignified old houses on gently curving, tree-lined streets. From here we'll make a vaguely triangular path that swings through the Kerns neighborhood's miniature Restaurant Row, along 28th Avenue, then down along a relatively unglamorous stretch of lower Sandy Boulevard that is home to a couple of storied, scruffy, well-loved dive bars. (Sensitive readers should note that there may be a small detour into nostalgia when we get to this part.) The third side of our lopsided triangle will be formed by East Burnside Street, one of the city's main east–west arteries and a constantly evolving business corridor, which among many other things is the site of an excellent second-run-movie theater and pub.

● Start at the bus stop at SE 39th Ave. (a.k.a. Cesar Chavez Blvd.) and Ash St. Take the paved path into the park toward the lake, following the part that veers off to the left. Laurelhurst Park covers about 26 acres and once belonged to William Ladd, the same former mayor responsible for Ladd's Addition (see Back Story: William S. Ladd on page 82). The park was designed in 1912, and in 2001 it became the first city park in the US to be listed on the National Register of Historic Places. The spring-fed central pond started out as a watering hole for cattle; for several years, an angry swan named General Pershing lorded over it. These days it's a great place to see baby ducks in spring (don't feed them). There are picnic spots scattered around, an off-leash dog run area, and gently hilly paved trails great for jogging. (Or, you know, walking.)

- Follow the path around the lake and on through the middle of the park until it bumps into SE 33rd Ave.; turn right onto 33rd. At the top of the short hill, turn left onto SE Ankeny St., then right at SE 32nd Ave. Where 32nd meets E. Burnside St., you'll find Music Millennium, an independent record store that has been a vital piece of the Portland music scene for decades (it was founded in 1969). Its larger outpost in Northwest Portland closed in 2007, but this location (the original) is still kicking, hosting frequent in-store performances and an annual Customer Appreciation BBQ.

- Turn left on E. Burnside and head down the hill. At NE 28th Ave., take a right. Between E. Burnside and NE Glisan Sts. along 28th is a strip of bars and restaurants of surprising range, from a small-plates wine bar to upscale diner food to gelato and gourmet chocolate. At the corner is Pambiche, whose vivid color scheme means you can't miss it; it's an always-packed, extremely cheerful Cuban restaurant.

- At NE Glisan St., turn left. For an incredibly glamorous version of the street you're now walking down, seek out indie-film director Aaron Katz's movie *Cold Weather,* shot in Portland; it makes Glisan St. and various other parts of the city seem lit from within, despite (or maybe because of) the gray skies and damp asphalt. The big brick apartment building on your left, called the Rasmussen, plays a pivotal role in *Cold Weather* (though it appears under an alias).

  There's a little curl at the end of Glisan St. where it meets NE 22nd Ave. and Sandy Blvd. Note the pawn shop at this corner. Until noise complaints from neighbors forced it to close in December 2000, this building held one of the all-time great rock clubs, EJ's—a grimy little den that rivaled Satyricon and LaLuna for the allegiance of the city's music scenesters in the 1990s. (EJ's was a strip club until 1994, when the owner switched to live music; neighbors made remarkably little fuss over *that* transformation.)

- On the other side of NE Sandy Blvd., at 21st Ave., you'll see a small, turreted stucco building that might once have been occupied by Smurfs. This is Club 21, where you'd go for cheap drinks between the bands at EJ's. It remains one of Portland's true dive bars, although new ownership has made a few improvements (the food is now far better than it needs to be, especially the burgers, and pinball has shoved aside the video-poker machines), taking care not to spoil its charm.

On a wall by the back door of Club 21, look for a framed black-and-white photo of historic Sandy Blvd. If you study it closely you'll notice a building shaped like a massive shoe. Until it was demolished, the Big Shoe—one of Sandy Blvd.'s many examples of mimetic architecture (it was a boot-repair shop originally)—stood in the lot next door to Club 21, now occupied by a credit union. Sadly, the only example left of this style of building is the Sandy Jug, which you can visit on Walk 20: Upper Sandy.

- Leaving Club 21, return to NE Sandy Blvd. and take a right. At NE 17th Ave. you'll come to See See Motor Coffee Co., an impeccably stylish coffee bar and motorcycle-friendly hangout-shop that's well worth venturing into (it sells Bell helmets, imported magazines, some outdoor apparel, rugged camping gear, and more). In one room there's a tool-lending program, which anyone who rides a vintage bike knows is pretty handy. Make sure you get a good look at the espresso machine, painted with psychedelic-wizard van art. See See also hosts frequent events, live music, parties, art shows, and so on—check their website for a schedule.

- Continue along NE Sandy Blvd. Where Sandy crosses NE Davis St. you'll see the Eastside outpost of Voodoo Doughnut, looking reliably hideous in its Pepto Bismol–lite color scheme (though much, much less crowded than its downtown sibling, in case you're desperate to tell folks back home that you tried a bacon-maple bar).

- Take a left at NE 15th Ave., just in front of the wedge-shaped Sandy Hut, another of the city's best (diviest? oldest? open-latest?) dive bars, similarly striking for its vivid hue. (In fairness, it has been repainted over the years and is now a little closer to blue than purple, but even so.) The Hut is a bar at which it's best to order a drink with two or fewer ingredients. Until recently its neon sign promised STEAMED CLAMS, but these, sadly, are no longer available. There's shuffleboard in the back, and on one wall is a fading but still lovely replica of an Al Hirschfeld drawing—entertain yourself by searching for the name Nina, which Hirschfeld hid in many of his pieces in honor of his daughter (there are supposedly three here, but your intrepid guides have only ever seen two).

- Dragging yourself reluctantly away from the Hut, continue along NE 15th Ave. and turn left on E. Burnside St. At NE 22nd Ave. you'll find one of Portland's coffee labs:

Heart Roasters, an industrial-chic hangout that opened in 2009 as part of the wave of post-Stumptown seriousness regarding the art and science of caffeination.

- Continue up E. Burnside St. to NE 28th Ave., home of the excellent Laurelhurst Theater. The Art Deco theater opened in 1923 as a single-screen movie house but now has several auditoriums and serves microbrews, wine, and pizza. It shows a handful of second-run films plus (usually) a classic or two selected by theme.

- Turn right on SE 28th Ave., then left on SE Ankeny St. Follow Ankeny past SE 33rd Ave. (where you exited the park earlier); glance to your right as you pass two old-Portland mansions looming on their small hillside. Stay on SE Ankeny St. until you reach the park entrance, just before SE Laurelhurst Pl., then take a right into the park. Follow the main path back through Laurelhurst Park to the starting point.

POINTS OF INTEREST (START TO FINISH)

Music Millennium musicmillennium.com, 3158 E. Burnside St., 503-231-8926

Pambiche pambiche.com, 2811 NE Glisan St., 503-233-0511

Club 21 2035 NE Glisan St., 503-235-5690

See See Motor Coffee Co. seeseemotorcycles.com, 1642 NE Sandy Blvd., 503-894-9566

Voodoo Doughnut Too voodoodoughnut.com, 1501 NE Davis St., 503-235-2666

The Sandy Hut sandyhut.com, 1430 NE Sandy Blvd., 503-235-7972

Heart Roasters heartroasters.com, 2211 E. Burnside St., 503-206-6602

Laurelhurst Theater laurelhursttheater.com, 2735 E. Burnside St., 503-232-5511

route summary

1. Start at SE Cesar Chavez Blvd. and Ash St.

2. Head into Laurelhurst Park, taking the path to the left.

3. Follow the path to SE 33rd Ave.

4. Turn right on SE 33rd Ave.

5. Turn left on SE Ankeny St.

6. Turn right on SE 32nd Ave.

7. Turn left on E. Burnside St.

8. Turn right on NE 28th Ave.

9. Turn left on NE Glisan St.

10. Cross NE Sandy Blvd. to NE 21st Ave.

11. From Club 21, turn right (southwest) on NE Sandy Blvd.

12. Turn left on NE 15th Ave.

13. Turn left on E. Burnside St.

14. Turn right on SE 28th Ave.

15. Turn left on SE Ankeny St.

16. Turn right, into Laurelhurst Park.

17. Follow park path back to starting point.

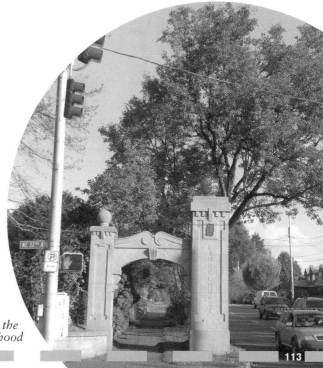

*One of the gates at the entrance to the
tony Laurelhurst neighborhood*

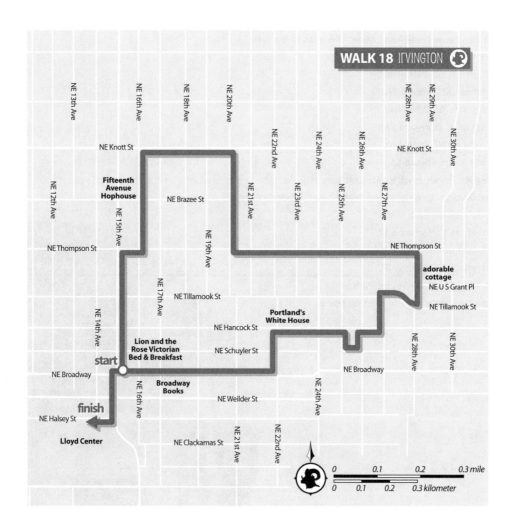

NE 13th Ave

NE 16th Ave

NE 18th Ave

NE 20th Ave

NE 22nd Ave

NE 24th Ave

NE 26th Ave

NE 28th Ave

NE 29th Ave

NE 30th Ave

NE Knott St

NE Knott St

NE 12th Ave

Fifteenth Avenue Hophouse

NE Brazee St

NE 21st Ave

NE 23rd Ave

NE 25th Ave

NE 27th Ave

NE 15th Ave

NE Thompson St

NE 19th Ave

NE Thompson St

adorable cottage

NE U S Grant Pl

NE 17th Ave

NE Tillamook St

NE Tillamook St

NE 14th Ave

Portland's White House

NE Hancock St

Lion and the Rose Victorian Bed & Breakfast

NE Schuyler St

NE 28th Ave

NE 30th Ave

start

NE Broadway

NE Broadway

NE Broadway

NE 16th Ave

Broadway Books

NE Weilder St

NE 24th Ave

finish

NE Halsey St

Lloyd Center

NE Clackamas St

NE 21st Ave

NE 22nd Ave

0   0.1   0.2   0.3 mile

0   0.1   0.2   0.3 kilometer

18 IRVINGTON: THE BEAUTIFUL AND THE DAMNED

BOUNDARIES: **NE Knott St., NE Weidler St., NE 15th Ave., NE 28th Ave.**
DISTANCE: **2.5 miles**
DIFFICULTY: **Easy**
PARKING: **Free street parking**
PUBLIC TRANSIT: **TriMet Bus 8 (NE 15th Ave. and Broadway), MAX Red and Blue Lines (Lloyd Center)**

Irvington was planned, successfully, as an upper-middle-class neighborhood, with strict rules about things like yard size and the proximity of sidewalks to front doors. There was also, for a long time, a rule against most commercial development, which in hindsight was a great idea, as it has allowed much of the neighborhood to be preserved as originally laid out: quiet, tree-lined streets with big, stately houses and well-landscaped yards. (This is not counting the parts that were demolished to build up the Lloyd District—more on that later.) Irvington is a pleasure to walk through, despite the lack of things to do here. This walk is mostly just a peaceful wander among the lovely old Victorian houses, with a couple of exceptions, and one jarring architectural and spiritual contrast that couldn't be avoided. (Spoiler alert: it's a mall.)

● Start the walk at the corner of NE 15th Ave. and Broadway. Head north along 15th. As you cross NE Schuyler St. you'll see an enormous sky-blue Queen Anne house, which is now Lion and the Rose Victorian Bed & Breakfast (fans of the NBC series *Grimm*, set and filmed in Portland, might recognize it from an episode in Season 1).

● Keep heading along NE 15th Ave. to NE Thompson St., where you'll turn right. Walk a block, then turn left onto NE 16th Ave. Follow 16th to NE Brazee St., where you have an opportunity for refreshment at the newly established Fifteenth Avenue Hophouse. Dozens of imported and craft beers are available here, along with some killer sweet-potato fries and other classed-up pub fare. It almost didn't open, which is surprising in light of its quiet, low-key, grown-up vibe. The Irvington Community Association voted in early 2011 not to grant the pub a liquor license, citing concerns about noise. (The president of the association told *The Oregonian* afterward that he thought the opposition was "generational.") That vote meant that the pub would be allowed to serve beer and wine but not be granted a full liquor license. But a "good-neighbor agreement" in the wake of the vote helped the two parties iron out their differences, and the pub opened with a full license and a lot of vocal support from neighbors.

- Continue along NE 16th Ave. to NE Knott St., and turn right. From Knott, take a right on NE 20th Ave. At NE Thompson St. turn left and continue several blocks, then turn right at NE 28th Ave.

- At the corner of NE 28th Ave. and U. S. Grant Pl. is an adorable cottage that stands out even in a neighborhood full of pretty houses. Note the extra-cool spiderweb window glass.

- Keep walking down NE 28th Ave. another block, then turn right onto NE Tillamook St. Go left at NE 27th Ave., then right onto NE Hancock St. for a block, then left onto NE 26th Ave., then right into the Hancock St.–Broadway Alley. Portland has a number of these unmaintained alleyways; they're public rights-of-way and open to (slow-moving) traffic, though often unpaved and challenging for cars. Mostly they're a fun way to see a neighborhood from a new angle: namely, the back door.

- Exiting the alley, take a right onto NE 25th Ave., then a left on NE Hancock St. At the corner of Hancock and NE 22nd Ave. is Portland's White House, a very sweet bed-and-breakfast in a historic, gorgeously renovated Victorian home.

- Turn left on NE 22nd, then right on NE Broadway, the neighborhood's main drag. You'll find any number of eating and drinking options along this stretch. Just before NE 17th Ave. is the excellent Broadway Books, an independent bookstore that holds frequent events and author appearances. The store is a particularly active supporter of regional authors, such as Chelsea Cain (*Heartsick*), Cheryl Strayed (*Wild*), and Storm Large (*Crazy Enough*). The staff is known for above-and-beyond customer service and maintains a fun blog, too (broadwaybooks.blogspot.com).

- Follow NE Broadway to NE 15th Ave., passing the route's starting point, crossing 15th and turning left. Turn right at NE Halsey (by the Applebee's, a harbinger if ever there was one), then left down the unlovely concrete path through the Lloyd Center mall parking lot.

Back Story: Oregon Convention Center

A few blocks southwest of the Lloyd Center mall is the Oregon Convention Center, easily spotted from anywhere near the river by its twin green-tinted glass spires. Opened in 1990 and renovated in 2003, the convention center encompasses almost a million square feet and covers the equivalent of 14–16 city blocks. It's owned by Metro (the regional government) and operated by a Metro subsidiary called MERC (Metropolitan Exposition Recreation Commission).

The convention center management prides itself on keeping the building green and energy-efficient; in 2004 the OCC became the first convention center anywhere to be awarded a LEED certification from the U.S. Green Building Council. It's filled with public art and interesting, practical features such as, for example, the rainwater garden in the southwest corner

of the center. The rainwater garden collects water from the roof of the building, then channels it along an artificial stream made to look like a real one, with native plants along its edges. Terraced pools slow down the water and filter out sediment; this system of treating the runoff saves the convention center around $15,000 a year, according to its website, and it reduces landscaping costs as well.

Public art in the building includes the world's largest bronze Foucault pendulum, weighing in at 900 pounds and 36 inches across; a 40-foot-long red dragon boat built in Taiwan, commemorating the dragon boat races held each year during Portland's Rose Festival; and the giant hanging sculpture *Gingkoberry Gwa* by New York City artist Ming Fay, with its enormous red-glass blossoms and gnarled roots.

Lloyd Center was a $100 million, 1.2-million-square-foot project when it opened in August 1960. (It was designed by architect John Graham, who also designed Seattle's Space Needle.) At the time it was considered a shining achievement in architecture, which is sort of astounding to contemplate when you look at it today. Of course, this was before the entire place was boxed in with a light-killing roof and, later, plastered end-to-end in grayish-beige carpet. The original design was for an open-air mall and community center, with fountains and sculptures amid the shops, large windows everywhere, and of course the crown jewel, a skating rink. (This rink, by the way, is one of the places where bad-girl Olympic figure skater–turned–boxer Tonya Harding used to practice.) In old photos, Lloyd Center actually does look quite attractive, with its water features and its airy spiral staircases lifting shoppers toward unlimited retail delights. But the mall was sold in 1986 and renovated to its present boxy status in 1990. (And by the way, in focusing on its terrible aesthetics, we're overlooking the mall's previous crimes: its construction involved the razing of several residential blocks, and its popularity helped sap downtown of its draw as a retail destination.) Love the skating rink, though.

● Back away slowly from the mall, turn left on NE 15th Ave., and retrace your steps up to NE Broadway to return to the walk's starting point.

POINTS OF INTEREST (START TO FINISH)

Lion and the Rose Victorian Bed & Breakfast lionrose.com, 1810 NE 15th Ave., 503-287-9245

Fifteenth Avenue Hophouse oregonhophouse.com, 1517 NE Brazee St., 971-266-8392

Portland's White House portlandswhitehouse.com, 1914 NE 22nd Ave., 503-287-7131

Broadway Books broadwaybooks.net, 1714 NE Broadway, 503-284-1726

Lloyd Center lloydcenter.com, 2201 Lloyd Center, 503-282-2511

route summary

1. Start at NE 15th Ave. & Broadway. Walk north on 15th.

2. Turn right on NE Thompson St.

3. Turn left on NE 16th Ave.

4. Turn right on NE Knott St.

5. Turn right on NE 20th Ave.

6. Turn left on NE Thompson St.

7. Turn right on NE 28th Ave.

8. Turn right on NE Tillamook St.

9. Turn left at NE 27th Ave.

10. Turn right on NE Hancock St.

11. Turn left on NE 26th Ave.

12. Turn right, into Hancock–Broadway Alley.

13. Turn right on NE 25th Ave.

14. Turn left on NE Hancock St.

15. Turn left on NE 22nd Ave.

16. Turn right on NE Broadway.

17. Cross NE 15th Ave. and turn left.

18. Turn right at NE Halsey St.

19. Turn left toward the entrance of Lloyd Center.

20. Turn left on NE 15th Ave. and retrace your steps to Broadway to return to the walk's starting point.

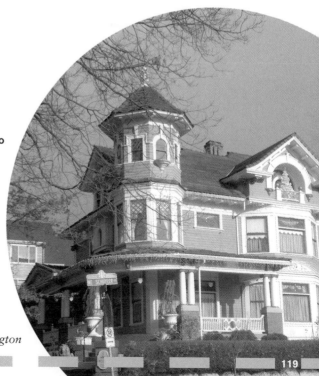

Lion and the Rose Victorian Bed & Breakfast in Irvington

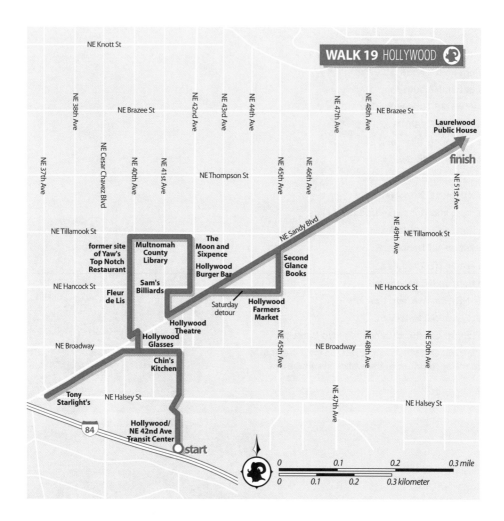

NE Knott St

WALK 19 HOLLYWOOD

NE 38th Ave

NE Brazee St

NE 42nd Ave

NE 43rd Ave

NE 44th Ave

NE 47th Ave

NE 48th Ave

NE Brazee St

Laurelwood
Public House

NE 37th Ave

NE Cesar Chavez Blvd

NE 40th Ave

NE 41st Ave

NE Thompson St

NE 45th Ave

NE 46th Ave

finish

NE 51st Ave

NE 49th Ave

NE Tillamook St

NE Sandy Blvd

NE Tillamook St

former site
of Yaw's
Top Notch
Restaurant

Multnomah
County
Library

The
Moon and
Sixpence

Hollywood
Burger Bar

Second
Glance
Books

NE Hancock St

Sam's
Billiards

NE Hancock St

Fleur
de Lis

Hollywood
Theatre

Saturday
detour

Hollywood
Farmers
Market

NE Hancock St

NE Broadway

Hollywood
Glasses

NE 45th Ave

NE Broadway

NE 48th Ave

NE 50th Ave

Chin's
Kitchen

NE 47th Ave

Tony
Starlight's

NE Halsey St

NE Halsey St

84

Hollywood/
NE 42nd Ave
Transit Center

start

0   0.1   0.2   0.3 mile

0   0.1   0.2   0.3 kilometer

19 HOLLYWOOD: aLMOST FaMOUS

BOUNDARIES: **NE 52nd Ave., NE Halsey St., NE 37th Ave., NE Brazee St.**
DISTANCE: **2 miles**
DIFFICULTY: **Easy**
PARKING: **Free street parking**
PUBLIC TRANSIT: **TriMet Bus 12 (NE 42nd Ave. and Sandy Blvd.), MAX Red and Blue Lines (Hollywood/NE 42nd Ave. Transit Center)**

Anchored by a fabulous old movie theater but otherwise pretty much unrelated to that other Hollywood, this is a fun little neighborhood that could be easily overlooked if you didn't know better. It's usually thought of as a place you go through on your way to somewhere else. MAX Light Rail has a stop here, adjacent to an important nexus of bus lines, so it's a key point for public transit. Plus, auto-worshiping Sandy Boulevard cuts right through the middle of it at a diagonal, and some of the resulting intersections will make you glad you're walking rather than driving. But overall the streets are mostly quiet and the atmosphere laid-back. It's a good in-between-things 'hood, close to several other parts of town, but Hollywood has come into its own as a destination in recent years. You'll want to stay awhile.

● Start at the Hollywood/NE 42nd Ave. Transit Center, where the MAX Light Rail line stops. Turn left (north) on the pedestrian bridge and continue straight along NE 42nd Ave. At NE Broadway, hang a left; note the excellent 1950s neon sign for Chin's Kitchen Chinese restaurant, on the left. Where Broadway meets NE Sandy Blvd., you'll see a yellow metal sculpture of a pair of vintage eyeglasses, lending its version of glamour to the neighborhood.

● Veer left onto NE Sandy and follow it a few blocks to where it meets NE Halsey St. For a few years in the early 2000s, the triangle-shaped corner building was home to The Blackbird, a short-lived but fondly remembered rock club of the sort that has all but disappeared, at least in Portland: small and cozy, with affordable door prices and zero pretension, but whose management was well-connected enough to book touring indie bands you'd actually heard of, bands that usually played much bigger venues. (It's now home to Tony Starlight's, a Vegas-style supper club and lounge that's one of the very few Portland venues with a dress code.)

Diagonally across Sandy is what used to be known as the 7-Up Building, although these days its bottle-shaped tower has a Budweiser sign where the 7-Up sign used to be. Before its decades-long run as the 7-Up Building (which lasted from the 1940s through 2002), this was the Steigerwald Dairy bottling plant, and the current cylindrical tower was actually milk-bottle-shaped. (The original bottle is still there, inside and underneath the cylinder, like a huge Russian nesting doll, and allegedly it can be glimpsed if you peek through the windows from the proper angle in just the right light.) The dairy opened in 1926 and was one of the first places to set up an automated bottling process. Its 75-foot-high tower was the tallest building in Portland for a while. The dairy closed in 1936, and the tower took on its new shape shortly thereafter.

● Backtrack up NE Sandy to NE 40th Ave., where you'll take a left over to NE Hancock St. At the corner is a great refueling spot inside the old public library building: Fleur de Lis, an artisan bakery run by Greg Mistell, who used to manage the Hollywood Farmers Market and, more to the point, once owned Pearl Bakery. It's very kid-friendly and is one of the few coffee shops in town without Wi-Fi, in case you're looking for a mini-vacation from technology. Try one of the enormous cinnamon rolls—*The Oregonian* called them the best in Portland, and they're surely the biggest—or a panini on rustic bread. The Fleur de Lis also supplies its bread to several of the city's best sandwich shops. Keep in mind that this is a popular neighborhood stop, so if you want the best selection of pastries, get here early.

● Keep going up NE 40th Ave. toward NE Tillamook St. On your left, where there is now a McDonald's, was the late, lamented Yaw's Top Notch Restaurant, a beloved drive-in burger joint that thrived during the sudden boom of car culture along Sandy Blvd. in the 1950s and '60s. Yaw's was one of the key stops for guys and dolls out cruisin' on a Saturday night. As the story goes, a traffic cop used to keep the wild youngsters in line by handing out Tootsie Rolls. Yaw's closed in 1982, after 56 years, but the owner and some of the original staff are planning to reopen it in another location, several blocks farther east in the Gateway neighborhood.

● At NE Tillamook St., turn right to pass the new Multnomah County Library; this branch is another example of the library's participation in innovatively designed multiuse buildings, incorporating shops and affordable living spaces to complement the structure's ostensible purpose.

● At NE 42nd Ave. take another right. Here you'll find one of the nicest European-style pubs in town: The Moon and Sixpence, with a great beer and whiskey selection, excellent fish-and-chips, darts, occasional acoustic music, authentically mauve carpet, and a huge back patio. If you didn't bring anything to read, you can borrow a battered volume from one of their crowded shelves.

● Continuing along NE 42nd Ave., you'll notice on the left another of the neighborhood's little nods to its namesake: a Hollywood-star sculpture–cum–bicycle rack at NE Hancock St. Turn right on Hancock, then left on NE 41st Ave., to admire the cheesy-but-charming murals gracing the exterior of Sam's Billiards. Sam's itself is a sort of disco-sleazy pool hall, well worth investigating if you're into that sort of thing (and who isn't, really?). Pool tables rent by the hour.

● Heading back toward Sandy Blvd., you'll see the impressive facade of the Hollywood Theatre. The Hollywood opened in 1926, back when a streetcar line ran up Sandy and this part of town was far enough away from downtown Portland to count as an excursion. The theater was an immediate hit. People showed up in droves, and the theater ended up giving the neighborhood its name (and, if you ask us, most of its enduring character, even today). The place struggled to hold on through the 1980s and '90s, but it was rescued in 1997 by Film Action Oregon, a nonprofit that has been gradually restoring the interior while transforming the place into an educational resource for film lovers. (See Back Story: Grindhouse Film Festival, next page.) It's one of the few cinemas left in town—or anywhere, really—that regularly shows movies on 35-mm film rather than in digital format, and the programming

The facade of the Hollywood Theatre

Back Story: GrinDhouse Film Festival

One of the coolest things about the Hollywood Theater is the Grindhouse Film Festival, which (though it started as an annual festival) is now an ongoing year-round series programmed by Dan Halsted, one of the Hollywood Theatre's programmers. Halsted has a vast collection of obscure, usually one-of-a-kind 35-mm prints of some of the craziest movies you've never heard of, as well as all the best and weirdest of the classic Hong Kong action films. He's a serious archivist, refreshingly free of irony—you don't go to Grindhouse screenings to feel all smarty-pants-cooler-than-the-movie; you go because the movies are sincerely awesome. (If you're familiar with the work of the Alamo Drafthouse, the Grindhouse Film Fest is along those same lines; Halsted and the Alamo guys are pals.) Halsted has recently become something of a celluloid-treasure hunter, traveling far and wide in search of lost and neglected movies—a few years ago he found a huge stash of vintage kung fu films stored beneath an old theater in Vancouver, BC, that had been closed since 1985.

Halsted screens something under the Grindhouse brand about once a week, and it's always worth checking out, though some of these lost treasures are better than others. (*Five Element Ninjas:* YES. *Miami Connection?* Well . . . yes, too, but maybe not for everybody.) He also does an annual (or thereabouts) evening of movie trailers from the 1970s and '80s that is surprisingly entertaining and wildly popular.

For details of what's coming up soon, check out **grindhousefilmfest.com**.

never fails to be interesting. (Now with beer!) It's all volunteer-run, and the organiza-tion's educational arm does things like putting pro-level equipment in the hands of talented young kids who want to make documentaries, or bringing animation classes to junior high schools, so you can feel good about springing for a ticket to see *The Thin Man* on the big screen with a pint of Laurelwood red ale on a Sunday afternoon.

● Turn left to continue up Sandy. At NE 42nd Ave. you'll see the very cute Hollywood Burger Bar, once upon a time a streetcar-ticket-sales office. It's a classic old-school burger joint from the 1950s, with a tiny lunch counter and a basic menu and little gold placards reserving some of the seats for regulars. Hours can be eccentric, but if it's open and you're hungry, stop in.

- If you're walking on a Saturday, take a right at NE Hancock St. and browse the busy Hollywood Farmers Market (May–October), in the parking lot between NE 44th and 45th Aves. It's one of the bigger and more established markets in Portland.

- Backtrack north (left) on NE 45th Ave. to return to Sandy. Continue right and up the hill, keeping an eye out for evidence of Portland's active medical-marijuana program among the various storefronts. Don't neglect a stop at Second Glance Books, a small independent bookshop with a selection that consists mostly of used paperbacks.

- Nearing the top of the hill is Laurelwood Public House, a great brewery with awesome beer that serves as a gathering spot for parents—it's known for being kid-friendly. If you don't happen to be kid-friendly yourself, a tiny balcony upstairs enables you to hide out with your pint and leave the Tater Tot set behind.

- From here you can choose to link with Walk 20: Upper Sandy or catch Bus 12 toward downtown, which stops at 42nd and Sandy, about a block from the bus/Light Rail station where the walk started.

POINTS OF INTEREST (START TO FINISH)

Fleur de Lis fleurdelisbakery.com, 3930 NE Hancock St., 503-459-4887

The Moon and Sixpence 2014 NE 42nd Ave., 503-288-7802

Sam's Billiards portlandpoolhall.com, 1845 NE 41st Ave.

Hollywood Theatre hollywoodtheatre.org, 4122 NE Sandy Blvd., 503-493-1128

Hollywood Burger Bar hollywoodburgerbar.com, 4211 NE Sandy Blvd., 503-288-6422

Hollywood Farmers Market hollywoodfarmersmarket.org, NE Hancock St. between 44th and 45th Aves.

Second Glance Books secondglancebooks.com, 4500 NE Sandy Blvd., 503-249-0344

Laurelwood Public House laurelwoodbrewpub.com, 5115 NE Sandy Blvd., 503-282-0622

route summary

1. Start at the Hollywood/NE 42nd Ave. Transit Center.
2. Take NE 42nd Ave. north from the pedestrian bridge.
3. Turn left on NE Broadway.
4. Veer left onto NE Sandy Blvd.
5. At NE Halsey St., turn around and retrace your path up NE Sandy Blvd.
6. Turn left at NE 40th Ave.
7. Turn right on NE Tillamook St.
8. Turn right on NE 42nd Ave.
9. Turn right on NE Hancock St.
10. Turn left on NE 41st Ave.
11. Turn left on NE Sandy Blvd.
12. Turn right on NE Hancock St.
13. Turn left on NE 45th Ave.
14. Turn right on NE Sandy Blvd.

connecting the walks

This walk can be extended to join Walk 20: Upper Sandy.

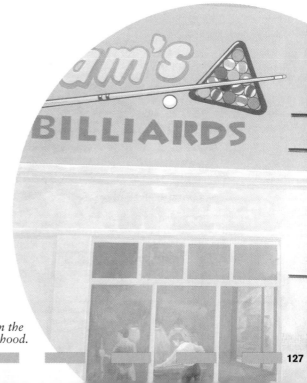

*Murals decorate Sam's Billiards, in the
Hollywood neighborhood.*

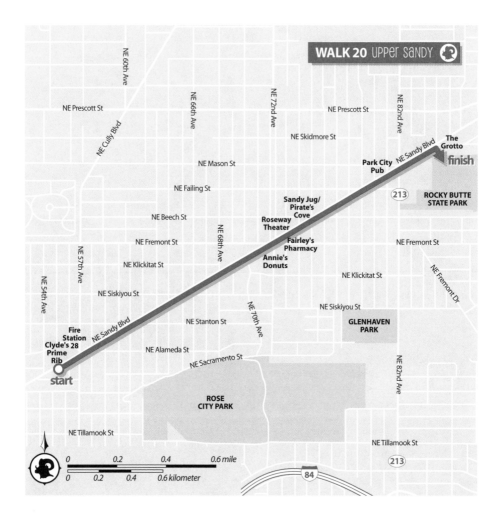

NE 60th Ave

NE 66th Ave

NE 72nd Ave

NE 82nd Ave

NE Prescott St

NE Prescott St

NE Cully Blvd

NE Skidmore St

The Grotto

finish

NE Mason St

Park City Pub

NE Sandy Blvd

NE Failing St

213

ROCKY BUTTE STATE PARK

Sandy Jug/ Pirate's Cove

NE Beech St

Roseway Theater

NE 68th Ave

NE Fremont St

Fairley's Pharmacy

NE Fremont St

NE 57th Ave

NE Klickitat St

Annie's Donuts

NE 54th Ave

NE Siskiyou St

NE Klickitat St

NE Fremont Dr

Fire Station

Clyde's 28 Prime Rib

NE Sandy Blvd

NE Stanton St

NE 70th Ave

NE Siskiyou St

GLENHAVEN PARK

start

NE Alameda St

NE Sacramento St

NE 82nd Ave

ROSE CITY PARK

NE Tillamook St

NE Tillamook St

213

| 0 | 0.2 | 0.4 | 0.6 mile |

| 0 | 0.2 | 0.4 | 0.6 kilometer |

84

20 upper sandy: Grotty to Grotto

BOUNDARIES: **NE 54th Ave., NE Sandy Blvd., NE Skidmore St.**
DISTANCE: **2 miles**
DIFFICULTY: **Easy**
PARKING: **Free street parking, lot at The Grotto**
PUBLIC TRANSIT: **TriMet Bus 12 (NE Sandy Blvd. and 54th Ave., NE Sandy Blvd. and The Grotto)**

Let's be up front about this: walking along Sandy Boulevard is unusual, unless you happen to work at one of a very limited number of occupations. It's not a street whose atmosphere is considered universally delightful. But it certainly has character, and it also has history. A lot of the things we'll point out on this walk don't exist anymore, but perhaps that's not so uncommon. The main thing to keep in mind is that Sandy Boulevard was invented for cars, in the age of automobile worship; in fact, it was so representative of this era that the Smithsonian Institution chose Sandy Boulevard for its permanent exhibit about automobile-oriented culture in the 1940s and '50s, under the title "Suburban Strip." (Yes, it also used to be considered suburban.) Walking up it, therefore, can be considered an exercise in shifting perspective. Relax and enjoy it.

● We'll dive right in and start this walk at NE 55th Ave. and Sandy Blvd., currently the location of Clyde's Prime Rib. Clyde's today is a fantastic old-school neighborhood steakhouse, with curving, high-backed booths in the dining room, red-velvet seats in the bar, many gigantic fireplaces, and an actual suit of shining armor guarding the main entrance. There's live music in the lounge most nights, and Clyde himself is often on hand, happily chatting with customers. But the restaurant's uncomfortable history adds another layer to the experience: from the 1930s to the 1950s, it was a restaurant called the Coon Chicken Inn, a fried-chicken joint whose name and logo consisted of what today are shocking racist stereotypes. The place closed when the owners retired in the 1950s and the staff realized that times had changed. (There were two other restaurants in the chain, one in Seattle and one in Salt Lake City, which both also shut down during the 1950s.)

● Half a block up NE Sandy Blvd. from Clyde's is the interestingly revamped Fire Station 28, originally built in 1913 as a barn, and renovated in 2005. The spiky, glowing sculpture in front of the building is called *Araminta: Carrying People to Safety*, by

Portland artist James M. Harrison; its title refers to the abolitionist Harriet Tubman (Araminta is the name she was given at birth).

- Continue up Sandy, stopping whenever the craving hits you at any of the great ethnic restaurants (mostly Thai and Vietnamese) along this stretch. Save room, though, for at least a couple of the truly excellent doughnuts at Annie's, just past SE 71st Ave., where Sandy meets NE Fremont St. There's no atmosphere to speak of here, but you won't need it: the doughnuts take care of everything. Get an apple fritter—for starters.

- Just across Fremont in a wedge-shaped building is Fairley's Pharmacy, which is cool not just for its geometrical architecture but also because it still has an old-fashioned soda fountain, with the counter and barstools and everything. Fairley's also appeared in Gus Van Sant's 1989 movie *Drugstore Cowboy*.

- Speaking of movies, just across the street is the single-screen Roseway Theater, one of the best of many excellent places to see a first-run movie in Portland. It has a killer sound system and a huge screen, plus loads of retro charm and popcorn that everyone says is the best in all of Portland. (Research on this last topic is still being conducted, but we have no real reason to doubt the claim.)

- A couple of blocks up Sandy, you'll come to a funny-looking bottle-shaped build-ing painted a disconcertingly murderous shade of red. This is the Sandy Jug, known these days as Pirate's Cove, and it's an example of the mimetic architecture that once made this street so much fun to cruise up and down. Basically, there used to be a lot of buildings on Sandy that were shaped like the thing they were selling. Originally built in 1928–29, the Jug has been an auto mechanic's shop, a café, a soda shop, a pool hall, and—for the past decade or so—a strip club. For years it was known both informally and officially as the Sandy Jug, but it seems to have embraced its new incarnation as Pirate's Cove with several nods to swashbuckler decor inside (and, it must be said, abundant booty).

- Pirate's Cove makes for a nice contrast with our next stop; luckily, you'll have plenty of time to walk off the sleaze before we get there. Continue up Sandy Blvd. for sev-eral blocks (noting, on your left at NE 80th Ave., the Park City Pub—this was once the steakhouse with the best name of any steakhouse ever: Sir Loins). Cross NE 82nd Ave. and continue a few more blocks until you see the entrance to The Grotto on your right (at about NE 85th Ave.). Go on in and follow signs to the visitors' entrance.

Officially called The National Sanctuary of Our Sorrowful Mother—you can see why the shorter moniker caught on—it's a 62-acre botanical garden surrounding a Catholic shrine. The actual grotto is a rock cave that was carved into the base of a hundred-foot cliff in 1923, with a replica of Michelangelo's *Pietà* nestled within it. Surrounding this are gardens on two levels, one of which is accessible by elevator (there's a fee for the lift, though). Wandering around The Grotto is a possibly disorienting experience for anyone coming directly from a walk down Sandy Blvd., but it's a quiet and calming pocket of nature and, if nothing else, a vivid juxtaposition.

● To return to your starting point, simply cross to the other side of Sandy Blvd. outside the entrance to The Grotto; you can catch TriMet Bus 12 at Sandy and NE 68th Ave.

POINTS OF INTEREST (START TO FINISH)

Clyde's Prime Rib clydesprimerib.com, 5474 NE Sandy Blvd., 503-281-9200

Fire Station 28 5540 NE Sandy Blvd.

Annie's Donuts 3449 NE 72nd Ave., 503-284-2752

Fairley's Pharmacy 7206 NE Sandy Blvd., 503-284-1159

Roseway Theater rosewaytheater.com, 7229 NE Sandy Blvd., 503-282-2898

Pirate's Cove piratescoveportland.com, 7417 NE Sandy Blvd., 503-287-8900

The Grotto thegrotto.org, NE 85th Ave. and Sandy Blvd., 503-254-7371

ROUTE SUMMARY

1. Start at NE 55th Ave. and Sandy Blvd.
2. Walk northeast up NE Sandy Blvd.
3. Cross NE 82nd Ave. to stay on Sandy.
4. Turn right to enter The Grotto.

CONNECTING THE WALKS

This route could be walked as a continuation of Walk 19: Hollywood.

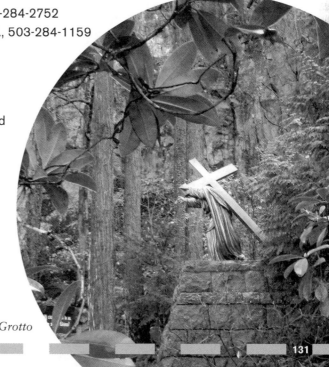

A sculpture near the entrance of The Grotto

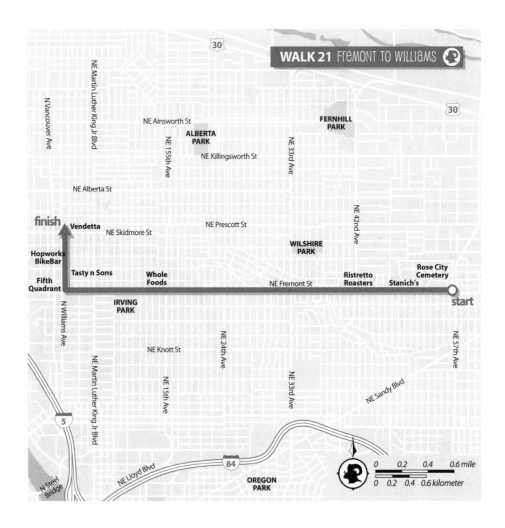

WALK 21 Fremont to Williams

30

30

NE Martin Luther King Jr Blvd

N Vancouver Ave

NE Ainsworth St

ALBERTA
PARK

NE 15th Ave

NE Killingsworth St

FERNHILL
PARK

NE 33rd Ave

NE Alberta St

NE 42nd Ave

finish

Vendetta

NE Skidmore St

NE Prescott St

WILSHIRE
PARK

Hopworks
BikeBar

Tasty n Sons

Whole
Foods

Ristretto
Roasters

Rose City
Cemetery

Fifth
Quadrant

NE Fremont St

Stanich's

start

IRVING
PARK

N Williams Ave

NE Martin Luther King Jr Blvd

NE Knott St

NE 24th Ave

NE 33rd Ave

NE 15th Ave

NE Sandy Blvd

NE 57th Ave

5

84

NE Lloyd Blvd

OREGON
PARK

0   0.2   0.4   0.6 mile
0   0.2   0.4   0.6 kilometer

N Steel
Bridge

21 FreMONT TO WILLIAMS: SHIFTING Gears

BOUNDARIES: **N. Williams Ave., NE Skidmore St., NE Fremont St., NE 50th Ave.**
DISTANCE: **3.5 miles**
DIFFICULTY: **Easy**
PARKING: **Free street parking**
PUBLIC TRANSIT: **TriMet Bus 44 (N. Williams Ave. and NE Skidmore St.) or Bus 24**
    (NE Fremont St. and 57th Ave.)

This walk starts at a lovely cemetery on top of a hill, then makes its way down the hill through various little hubs of commercial activity, most of which have sprung up fairly recently. The walk concludes with a stretch of funky Williams Avenue, a major bicycle corridor busy with new commercial development that's been drawing some of the most talked-about buildings and businesses in town. (The nature of this development has been strongly influenced by the fact that there's so much bicycle traffic along here; the two things have been feeding each other. If you've been curious about the much-hyped Portland bike culture, the Williams Avenue corridor is a good place to get an up-close look at it.) This is definitely an area in flux: if you walk it now, try walking it again in six months— we bet you'll see big changes.

● Start at the bus stop at NE Fremont St. and 57th Ave., next to the extremely beautiful Rose City Cemetery (established in 1906). In the middle of the main cemetery is a separate, enclosed Japanese Cemetery. Go in for a look, or simply wander down Fremont alongside the quiet, atmospheric grounds.

● At NE 52nd Ave. you'll reach a small cluster of eateries and coffee shops, including Stanich's, known for its enormous burgers. George and Gladys Stanich opened the joint in 1949. Gladys cooked, and George became known as "The Philosopher of Fremont." The place is jam-packed with sports memorabilia, team pennants, and good vibes.

● Around NE 42nd Ave. and Fremont is the tiny hub of Beaumont Village, which is essentially just a small neighborhood market (in a building called the Swiss House—

you'll recognize it), a handful of shops and cafés, and a very tiny but very good espresso bar, Ristretto Roasters, just off Fremont to the right.

● Continue west along what is now mostly residential Fremont St. for several blocks. At the bottom of a long hill, by NE 15th Ave., is another hub of commercial activity, centered around a Whole Foods grocery store. In the next block are two good pubs and a coffee shop—hard to go wrong.

● Keep walking along Fremont until you reach Irving Park on your left, just past NE 11th Ave. This hilly, shady park is a great place to wander around or to bust out any picnic supplies you may have collected at the grocery store a few blocks back. (The park is named after an ancient mariner, or, rather, a sea captain who had a land claim here in Portland's early days.)

● Stay on Fremont St. for several more blocks, crossing NE Martin Luther King Jr. Blvd. at the traffic signal and continuing on. At N. Williams Ave., turn right. Williams is one of the major north–south thoroughfares for bicycle traffic (note the nice wide bike lanes along this street). Nearly 3,000 cyclists commute along this corridor daily. A block or so farther along, the building on the right, between Beech and Failing Sts. on Williams, is currently home to some of the best-loved eateries and drinkeries in Portland, including Tasty n Sons restaurant. It's run by the same chef who established the deeply loved Toro Bravo, and it was chosen as *Willamette Week*'s Restaurant of the Year in 2010. There's nearly always a huge line, so get here early if you're interested in a table, especially at brunch. If you missed the chance for an espresso earlier, there's another Ristretto Roasters here.

This building, called The Hub, was conceived as a European-style marketplace and renovated as such in 2008; in addition to Tasty n Sons and several other small businesses, its tenants include a naturopathic veterinarian, a yoga studio, and a restaurant that serves mainly oysters. Call it gentrification if you will—that's pretty much what it is—but whatever, it's a lovely building, and frankly it's hard to imagine complaining over a bowl of Tasty n Sons' Burmese red-pork stew.

● Across the street is another good eating and drinking place, and an early arrival to this neighborhood: the Fifth Quadrant pub. It's run by Lompoc Brewing, so it serves the familiar and well-loved Lompoc brews, but the food is a little more sophisticated here, and the room itself is all blonde wood and honeyed lighting. Next door there's a tasting room, the Sidebar, where you can sample specialty beers that aren't available anywhere else. This is also the place to pick up a keg or a few bottles to go.

- Continuing along N. Williams Ave., you'll pass any number of shops, bars, and restaurants, and probably twice as many as there were at the time this was written—the neighborhood has definitely been discovered. Try anything that looks interesting! There's a bicycle-themed brewpub on the left, run by Hopworks Urban Brewery, with custom bike frames hung over the bar, a water-bottle filling station, and a range of organic microbrews on tap. The brewpub occupies the ground floor of a new apartment building, called ecoFLATS, which is designed around sustainability, bike-friendliness, low energy use, and beer. (There's a flat-screen TV monitor in the entryway to the apartments that displays the amount of energy consumption for each tenant, in real time. Motivating!) The building's appearance is in line with several other new apartment blocks of recent vintage: sleek and square, with slightly weathered-looking and reclaimed materials whose rough textures provide an appealing contrast with the building's precise shapes and clean lines. It's a good look, although it's hard to say if the style will age well.

- A little farther along, at the corner of N. Williams and NE Skidmore St., you'll find the very friendly and comfortable Vendetta, a totally unpretentious hangout of a bar with a large, covered patio and a pair of garage-style main doors that are kept open in warm weather. There's a shuffleboard table and usually really good local art on the walls. Overall the place has the settled, established feel of a beloved neighborhood spot that makes it a nice anchor for this rapidly growing, changing area.

- To return to the starting point, retrace your steps back to NE Fremont St. and catch Bus 24 heading east.

POINTS OF INTEREST (START TO FINISH)

Rose City Cemetery 5625 NE Fremont St.

Stanich's stanichs.com, 4915 NE Fremont St., 503-281-2322

Ristretto Roasters ristrettoroasters.com, 3520 NE 42nd Ave., 503-284-6767

Tasty n Sons tastynsons.com, 3808 N. Williams Ave., 503-621-1400

Fifth Quadrant lompocbrewing.com, 3901 N. Williams Ave., 503-288-3996

Hopworks BikeBar hopworksbeer.com, 3947 N. Williams Ave., 503-287-6258

Vendetta vendettapdx.com, 4306 N. Williams Ave., 503-288-1085

ROUTE SUMMARY

1. Start at NE Fremont St. and 57th Ave.
2. Walk west along NE Fremont St.
3. Turn right at N. Williams Ave.
4. Walk ends at N. Williams Ave. and NE Skidmore St.

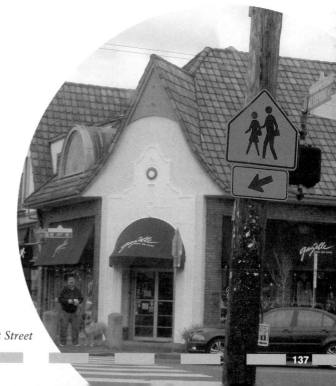

Beaumont Village, along NE Fremont Street

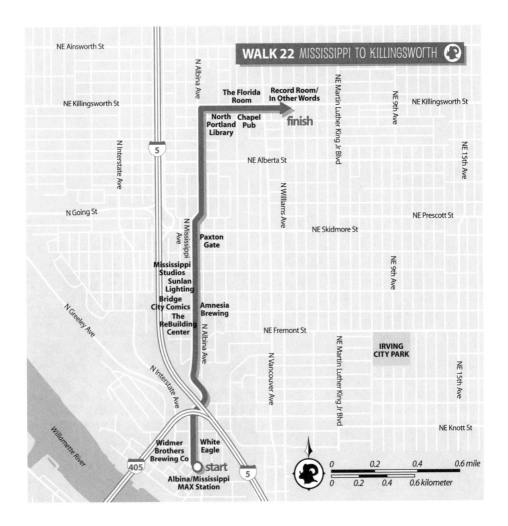

WALK 22 MISSISSIPPI TO KILLINGSWORTH

NE Ainsworth St

NE Killingsworth St

N Albina Ave

The Florida Room

Record Room/ In Other Words

NE Martin Luther King Jr Blvd

NE 9th Ave

NE Killingsworth St

North Portland Library

Chapel Pub

finish

5

NE Alberta St

N Interstate Ave

N Williams Ave

NE 15th Ave

N Going St

NE Prescott St

N Mississippi Ave

Paxton Gate

NE Skidmore St

NE 9th Ave

Mississippi Studios

Sunlan Lighting

Bridge City Comics

The ReBuilding Center

Amnesia Brewing

N Albina Ave

NE Fremont St

NE Martin Luther King Jr Blvd

N Greeley Ave

IRVING CITY PARK

NE 15th Ave

N Vancouver Ave

N Interstate Ave

NE Knott St

Willamette River

Widmer Brothers Brewing Co

White Eagle

start

405

Albina/Mississippi MAX Station

5

0   0.2   0.4   0.6 mile

0   0.2   0.4   0.6 kilometer

MISSISSIPPI TO KILLINGSWORTH: UPWARDLY MOBILE

BOUNDARIES: **NE Killingsworth St., N. Mississippi Ave., N. Tillamook St., Martin Luther King Jr. Blvd.**
DISTANCE: **2 miles**
DIFFICULTY: **Moderate**
PARKING: **Free street parking**
PUBLIC TRANSIT: **TriMet Bus 6 (NE Martin Luther King Jr. Blvd. and NE Killingsworth St.),
MAX Yellow Line (Albina/Mississippi Station)**

The Mississippi neighborhood is one of the more recently reinvigorated (or gentrified, if you must) parts of town. Walking through it still brings the excitement of discovery, and though it's not exactly rough around the edges anymore, it nevertheless preserves its past, often in the form of lovingly restored buildings with wholly new functions. With this walk, we follow North Mississippi Avenue from end to end and then join up with North Killingsworth Street, one of Northeast Portland's main thoroughfares.

● Start at the Albina/Mississippi MAX Station. From here, turn right onto N. Mississippi Ave. One block up, N. Russell St. is worth a one-block side trip in either direction: to the left you'll find Widmer Brewing Company, one of Portland's pioneering brew-pubs, housed in a former theater building; to the right (uphill) is one of the local McMenamin Brothers' more agreeable properties, the White Eagle. Once upon a time, the White Eagle was a fairly disreputable hotel and rowdy dock-worker drinking establishment, nicknamed the Bucket of Blood for its frequent and messy bar brawls. These days it's a perfectly civilized bar-restaurant with live country-folk music most nights. It's supposed to be haunted, so stay alert. (There are also hotel rooms upstairs, if you're thinking of staying awhile.)

● But don't get sidetracked for too long; we're just getting started. Continue straight ahead along N. Mississippi Ave., following the S-curve of the road as it passes beneath the I-5 and I-405 overpasses. It's a fairly steep climb to the top of the hill, but the path flattens out just past N. Fremont St.

● Halfway down the block on your left is The ReBuilding Center, a cool idea in a cool space: it's a nonprofit that gathers used building materials (from demolitions, donations, and the like) that might otherwise have been thrown out, then sells them as part of a sustainable-building effort. Far from the cookie-cutter stuff you might find at an ordinary retail store, the fixtures and frames and various odds and ends here are unique enough that it's fun just to browse. There's an "idea library" for those seeking inspiration. And the building itself embodies the principles in which it trades: it's a funky hodgepodge of salvaged material that somehow looks just right when put together.

● At the corner of N. Beech St. and Mississippi Ave., on the right, is one of the more appealing brewpubs in town, Amnesia Brewing. It's best in warm weather, when you can sit on the patio with a pint and a bratwurst in a bun and watch the traffic go by.

● Diagonally across the street from Amnesia Brewing is Bridge City Comics, a fine, friendly, and completely unintimidating comic-book shop, known for the well-attended author events and readings it hosts.

● As you continue along N. Mississippi, note Sunlan Lighting on your left, at N. Failing St. The shop itself is only mildly odd, but the commercials it used to run on late-night TV were of such a particular degree of bizarre that any local who has lived here long enough to have seen them will know exactly what you're talking about when asked. (Incidentally, it's a great place to find lightbulbs in unusual sizes, should you need any.)

● A few doors down is Mississippi Studios, a small live-music venue, and its attached watering hole, called Bar Bar. The venue is intimate and impeccably booked, with a sort of tiny-screening-room feel plus a balcony, and the bar serves awesome burgers that start at just $5 (no kidding). Alert walkers may also notice that the bar's outdoor patio makes use of materials from The ReBuilding Center down the street. This is definitely one of the best places to see a band (or just hang out and grab a bite), but get there early, because it does fill up.

● Farther along N. Mississippi is Paxton Gate, a store that is almost more of a taxi-dermy museum. (The original location, in San Francisco, started out as a gardening store, but it took off in an unexpected direction fairly soon.) It bills itself as a shop for "Treasures and Oddities," a place to find things for your personal wonder-cabinet: fossils, bones, teeth and eyes, adorable terrariums, etchings, mysterious items in jars, and, of course, the odd gardening implement. Definitely worth a look around, and the interior of the store itself is beautiful too.

● At N. Prescott St., Mississippi kinks to the right and becomes N. Albina Ave. Make your way along Albina for several blocks until you reach N. Killingsworth St.; turn right on Killingsworth.

● Just past N. Commercial Ave. on Killingsworth St. is a very turquoise dive bar called The Florida Room, famous for its Bloody Marys. Across the street is the Chapel Pub, a cute little building originally from 1932, now yet another in the string of drinkeries in repurposed buildings owned by the local McMenamins chain.

● Back on the other side of the street is the North Portland branch of the county library—originally the Carnegie Library, built in 1913. It was restored in 1999 and looks fantastic inside and out.

● At the corner of NE Killingsworth St. and N. Williams Ave. are a pair of shops whose customer overlap would be interesting to study: first there's In Other Words, a feminist bookstore that's been skewered on *Portlandia,* and then next door is the Record Room, an indie record store where you can enjoy beer, wine, coffee, and pinball while you browse through the new and used LPs and cassingles. If it hasn't already had its 15 minutes of *Portlandia* fame, it surely will in the very near future.

● Retrace your steps to N. Albina Ave., then catch Bus 4 back toward the city center and your starting point.

POINTS OF INTEREST (START TO FINISH)

Widmer Brothers Brewing Company widmerbrothers.com/brewery, 929 N. Russell St., 503-281-2437

White Eagle mcmenamins.com/whiteeaglesaloon, 836 N. Russell St., 503-282-6810

The ReBuilding Center rebuildingcenter.org, 3625 N. Mississippi Ave., 503-331-1877

Amnesia Brewing amnesiabrews.com, 832 N. Beech St., 503-281-7708

Bridge City Comics bridgecitycomics.com, 3725 N. Mississippi Ave., 503-282-5484

Sunlan Lighting sunlanlighting.com, 3901 N. Mississippi Ave., 503-281-0453

Mississippi Studios and Bar Bar mississippistudios.com, 3939 N. Mississippi Ave., 503-288-3895

Paxton Gate paxtongatepdx.com, 4204 N. Mississippi Ave., 503-719-4508

The Florida Room 435 N. Killingsworth St., 503-287-5658

Chapel Pub mcmenamins.com/chapel, 430 N. Killingsworth St., 503-286-0372

North Portland Library multcolib.org, 512 N. Killingsworth St., 503-988-5394

In Other Words inotherwords.org, 14 NE Killingsworth St., 503-232-6003

Record Room recordroompdx.com, 8 NE Killingsworth St., 971-544-7685

route summary

1. Start at the Albina/Mississippi MAX Station.
2. Turn right on N. Mississippi Ave.
3. At N. Prescott St. jog right, onto N. Albina Ave.
4. Turn right on N. Killingsworth St.

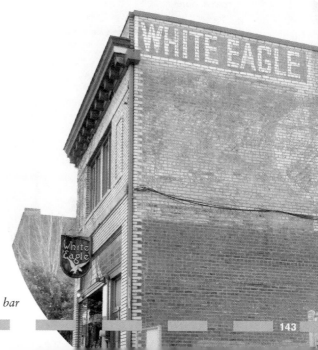

The once-rowdy White Eagle bar

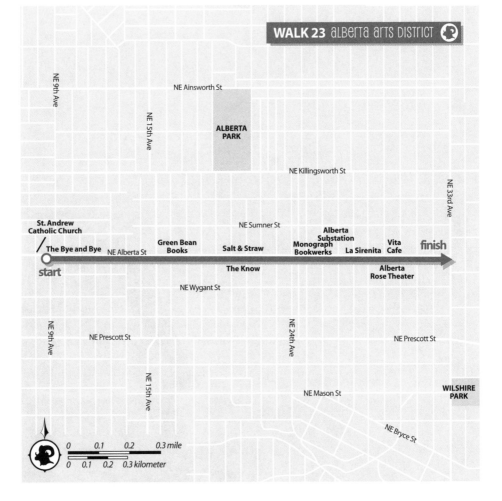

WALK 23 alberta arts district

NE 9th Ave

NE Ainsworth St

NE 15th Ave

ALBERTA PARK

NE Killingsworth St

NE 33rd Ave

St. Andrew Catholic Church

NE Sumner St

Alberta Substation

The Bye and Bye   NE Alberta St   Green Bean Books   Salt & Straw   Monograph Bookwerks   La Sirenita   Vita Cafe   finish

start   The Know   Alberta Rose Theater

NE Wygant St

NE 9th Ave

NE Prescott St

NE 24th Ave

NE Prescott St

NE 15th Ave

NE Mason St

WILSHIRE PARK

NE Bryce St

0   0.1   0.2   0.3 mile
0   0.1   0.2   0.3 kilometer

23 alberta arts district: artisan living

BOUNDARIES: NE 33rd Ave., NE 9th Ave., NE Alberta St.
DISTANCE: 1.25 miles
DIFFICULTY: Easy
PARKING: Free street parking
PUBLIC TRANSIT: TriMet Bus 72 (NE Alberta St. and 9th Ave.), Bus 70 (NE Alberta St. and 33rd Ave.)

If you'd left Portland in the early 1990s and not heard a word about it since, you would be astounded by the changes that have since taken place along NE Alberta Street. Back then, more than half of the businesses were shuttered, and nobody yet was using the term *gentrification* anywhere near here. But things change quickly. As is ever the way, bold artistic types noticed the cheap rent and made their way over, hipsters and hangers-on soon followed, and then came the business dollars, the building renovations, the local press's guilt-ridden griping about forcing longtime locals out of the neighborhood, followed by still more emboldened newcomers . . . you know the story.

These days the district is settling into its comfortably gentrified role; the identity crises seem mostly to have passed. It's now considered one of the most desirable neighborhoods in Portland, and it boasts a thriving arts scene that has matured significantly since its early days of silly posthippie summer-camp crafting displays. The last Thursday of each month, Alberta turns into a chaotic street fair that has only nominally to do with artists and art galleries. Thousands of people attend—don't plan on driving or parking anywhere near here on those evenings. It's well worth seeing, though, even if it's not necessarily everyone's cup of tea. If street fairs aren't your thing, don't despair: this part of town easily holds its own any day of the week.

● **Start at the bus stop at NE Alberta St. and 9th Ave. From here you can see the land-mark French Gothic towers of St. Andrew Catholic Church. This spot has been home to a chapel since 1907, when a group of Irish immigrants pooled their resources and bought the land. It's known today as a diverse and open-minded organization, reflecting the character of the neighborhood.**

● **Head east on NE Alberta. Wander up a block or so until you reach NE 10th Ave., where on your left you'll see The Bye and Bye, a great bar and restaurant with** awesome mason-jar drinks and a menu of Southern comfort food that just happens to be entirely vegan. The space is beautiful, and the crowd tends to be as well.

- At NE 15th Ave. is Green Bean Books, an excellent children's bookstore the likes of which every kid ought to have the chance to explore at some point. There are all kinds of nooks and crannies to cozy up in, plus fun little gifts, a summertime garden and deck, and regular events, including author readings, crafts nights, and multi-lingual storytime sessions.

- Continue up the street until you reach about NE 20th Ave., at which point you'll begin to smell the heavenly sweetness that is Salt & Straw. This newish artisan-ice-cream shop (which started out as a tiny mobile cart, like many other successful Portland food ventures) has quickly become an obsession for locals and tourists alike; you could call it the new Voodoo Doughnut (but no Crunch Berries on anything, as far as we know, and nothing anatomically shaped). People stand in line for ages to get their hands on a scoop or two of the salted caramel, or the balsamic strawberry, or the honey lavender. At first glance this seems ridiculous, lining up around the block to wait for ice cream, until you taste the stuff. OK, even then it's a little bit ridiculous, but we dare you to try walking blithely past the front door once you catch a whiff of this place. (Another location, on NW 23rd Ave., has equally long lines.)

- Across the street from Salt & Straw is one of the more under-the-radar clubs in Portland: The Know. It's a divey, no-frills, Pabst-in-a-can type of place with pinball and live-rock shows and cool bartenders. There are about a thousand other places on Alberta to get a drink, but this is probably the one where you're least likely to worry about what label you're wearing or whether you can afford a second round.

- At NE 27th Ave., duck around the corner to the left to find Monograph Bookwerks, a fine-art bookstore owned by a couple of artists, one of whom also owns Le Happy, a crêpes restaurant in the Northwest Portland neighborhood of Slabtown. The shop sells rare and small-press art books, plus a carefully chosen selection of prints, objects, and supplies.

- Across NE 27th Ave. from the bookshop you'll see the revamped Northwestern Electric Company Alberta Substation, built in 1931 but drastically renovated in 2005. What was once an unvarnished concrete labyrinth (with loads of grimy atmosphere, we might add) is now a spacious, attractive space that most recently held an upscale Thai restaurant and lounge, Siam Society. It's worth looking inside to see the transformation.

- Continuing along Alberta, just beyond NE 28th Ave. you'll come to La Sirenita, which for a very long time was pretty much the only place to get a decent taco or burrito within the city limits. These days the options are practically unlimited, but La Sirenita gets props for being here first.

- A movie house from 1927 until 1978, the Alberta Rose Theatre at NE 30th Ave. was closed for 20 years until it reemerged as a 300-seat live-music venue. It's also where the very worthwhile *Live Wire!* radio program is recorded in front of an audience (visit livewireradio.org for more info).

- Opened in 1999, Vita Cafe was part of the vanguard of both the Alberta restaurant scene and the wave of vegan-vegetarian dining options in Portland. This was in the era before anyone had given much thought to gluten, pro or con, and tofu was generally considered a form of punishment. The Vita dedicated itself to using sustainable business practices and became a leader in thoughtful restaurant dining, all the while churning out meals that made healthy eating taste good. The staff worked with locally and organically produced ingredients, and the restaurant dedicated a percentage of sales to environmental nonprofits. Some people might have found these practices a little stuffy at the time, or at least intimidatingly pure-hearted, but these days it just seems like ordinary good behavior. Progress!

- NE Alberta St. is so densely packed with things to look at that the best way to return to the starting point is simply to retrace your steps. If you're tired, though, you can also catch Bus 72.

POINTS OF INTEREST (START TO FINISH)

St. Andrew Catholic Church standrewchurch.com, 806 NE Alberta St., 503-281-4429

The Bye and Bye thebyeandbye.com, 1011 NE Alberta St., 503-281-0537

Green Bean Books greenbeanbookspdx.com, 1600 NE Alberta St., 503-954-2354

Salt & Straw saltandstraw.com, 2035 NE Alberta St., 503-208-3867

The Know theknowbar.com, 2026 NE Alberta St., 503-473-8729

Monograph Bookwerks monographbookwerks.com, 5005 NE 27th Ave., 503-284-5005

Alberta Substation 2703 NE Alberta St.

La Sirenita 2817 NE Alberta St., 503-335-8283

Alberta Rose Theatre albertarosetheatre.com, 3000 NE Alberta St., 503-719-6055

Vita Cafe vita-cafe.com, 3023 NE Alberta St., 503-335-8233

ROUTE SUMMARY

1. Start at NE Alberta St. and 9th Ave.
2. Walk east on NE Alberta St.
3. Walk ends at Alberta St. and NE 33rd Ave.

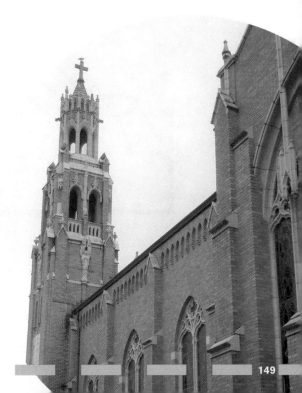

St. Andrew Catholic Church, on NE Alberta Street

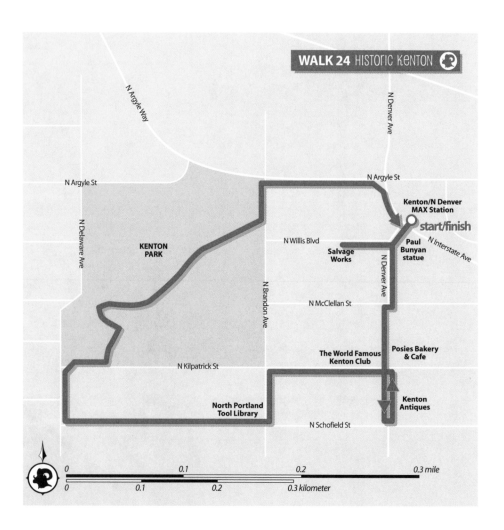

Kenton/N Denver
MAX Station

start/finish

N Argyle Way

N Argyle St

N Denver Ave

N Delaware Ave

KENTON
PARK

N Willis Blvd

Salvage
Works

Paul
Bunyan
statue

N Interstate Ave

N Brandon Ave

N Denver Ave

N McClellan St

Posies Bakery
& Cafe

The World Famous
Kenton Club

N Kilpatrick St

Kenton
Antiques

North Portland
Tool Library

N Schofield St

| 0 | | 0.1 | | 0.2 | | 0.3 mile |
| 0 | 0.1 | | 0.2 | | 0.3 kilometer | |

BOUNDARIES: N. Columbia Blvd., I-5, N. Chautauqua Blvd., N. Lombard St.
DISTANCE: 1 mile
DIFFICULTY: Easy
PARKING: Free street parking
PUBLIC TRANSIT: TriMet MAX Yellow Line (Kenton/N. Denver Station)

Historic Kenton is a funky little out-of-the-way part of town that has a no-nonsense, totally unpretentious center and an interesting past. Kenton began as a company town in 1911, founded by the Swift Meat Packing Company. These days it might be best known as the home of former Portland Mayor Sam Adams. The area has benefited recently from a $2.85 million "greenscaping" and revitalization program courtesy of the Portland Development Commission and the city's Bureau of Transportation. New businesses and shopfronts have been moving in, and young barflies have been known to travel from the depths of Southeast Portland to see indie bands play at Kenton watering holes. Plus it has its own branch of the Portland Farmers Market now (at North Denver Avenue and McClellan Street). Kenton's most famous landmark (despite the charming bravado of the World Famous Kenton Club) is the giant Paul Bunyan statue at the intersection of North Interstate and Denver Avenues, near the MAX station; it's a relic from the Oregon Centennial celebrations in Kenton in 1959.

● Start at the Kenton/N. Denver MAX Station and walk across N. Interstate Ave. to the giant Paul Bunyan lumberjack statue. He's 35 feet tall and was put here in 1959 to welcome folks who came to Portland for the Oregon Centennial Exposition, but now he serves primarily to set an example for fashion trends among the young men of the Portland area. (Just kidding. Mostly.)

● Follow N. Denver Ave. straight (southwest), then cross N. Willis Blvd., heading right (west). Walk about halfway down the block, and on your left you'll find Salvage Works, which now shares its space with Solabee Flowers and the very cool former pop-up shop Boys Fort. Salvage Works has all kinds of vintage building materials, and Boys Fort is sort of a shop for grown-up Eagle Scouts, a hodgepodge of the kind of knick-knacks and antiques that appeal to men (who knew there was such a thing?), plus handmade gifts, found objects, and vintage odds and ends of various sorts.

- Walk back along N. Willis Blvd. to return to N. Denver Ave., and turn right. At N. McClellan St., cross to the other side of N. Denver and continue the way you were going (south), past several friendly neighborhood watering holes. Follow Denver for a couple of blocks until you get to Posies Bakery & Cafe, where you should definitely go in and have a scone or a sandwich. This is a tiny, lovely, locally owned, kid-friendly community hangout with great coffee and baked treats, and rotating displays of art-work on the walls. The café is part of the monthly Third Thursday Art Walk in Kenton.

  The empty brown building between Posies and the new Multnomah County Library branch is a sore point with many Kenton residents. It's owned by former NBA guard Terrell Brandon, who has apparently done nothing with it since he bought it in 2001. An *Oregonian* article reported that homeless people were squatting in the building, which hasn't done much to put neighbors at ease.

- Continue another block or so along N. Denver Ave. and you'll come to Kenton Antiques. A labor of love run by a woman who left the corporate world to buy the place a few years ago, the store has all kinds of goodies, from furniture to Pez dispensers.

- When you reach the corner of N. Denver Ave. and Schofield St., cross Denver and turn around, walking back up to N. Kilpatrick St. on the other side of the street. Take a left on Kilpatrick. Half a block in is the (deservedly, although not actually) World Famous Kenton Club, an excellent lowbrow hangout with a rocky facade, a wood-paneled inte-rior, cheap drinks, live music, and a friendly, rowdy crowd.

- Take N. Kilpatrick St. to N. Brandon Ave. and turn left. At N. Schofield St. take a right. On this corner is the Historic Kenton Firehouse, home to the North Portland Tool Library. The Tool Library does just what you'd imagine: it lends tools, free of charge, to neighborhood residents who need to use them but might not want (or be able) to buy their own. (Seriously, how often are you really going to use a belt sander? Wouldn't it make more sense just to borrow one?) It also holds regular hands-on workshops (free of charge) so people can learn how to use the tools they're borrowing.

- Follow N. Schofield St. until you get to N. Delaware Ave., and turn right. Veer right again, just before N. Halleck St., to enter Kenton Park. A paved pathway steers you diagonally through the center of the park; a children's playground is off to the left. On a hot day, seek out the awesome "spraypark," which takes running through the sprinklers to a whole new level.

● At the far (northeast) corner of the park, you'll come to N. Argyle St. and turn right. Veer right at N. Interstate Ave. to return to the starting point and good old Paul Bunyan.

POINTS OF INTEREST (START TO FINISH)

Salvage Works, Boys Fort, Solabee Flowers salvageworkspdx.com, 2030 N. Willis Blvd., 503-285-2555

Posies Bakery & Cafe posiescafe.com, 8208 N. Denver Ave., 503-289-1319

Kenton Antiques kentonantiquespdx.com, 8112 N. Denver Ave., 503-490-8855

The World Famous Kenton Club kentonclub.com, 2025 N. Kilpatrick St., 503-285-3718

North Portland Tool Library northportlandtoollibrary.org, 2209 N. Schofield St., 503-823-0209

Kenton Park 8417 N. Brandon Ave.

ROUTE SUMMARY

1. Start at the Kenton/N. Denver MAX Station.
2. Cross N. Interstate Ave. to the Paul Bunyan statue.
3. Go straight along N. Denver Ave., then turn right across Denver to N. Willis Blvd.
4. Retrace your steps to N. Denver Ave. and turn right.
5. At N. McClellan St., cross to the other side of N. Denver, still heading right (south).
6. At N. Schofield St., recross N. Denver and turn right.
7. Turn left on N. Kilpatrick St.
8. Turn left on N. Brandon Ave.
9. Turn right on N. Schofield St.
10. Turn right on N. Delaware Ave.
11. Veer right, into Kenton Park.
12. Follow pathway through the park.
13. At N. Argyle St., exit park and turn right.
14. Veer right at N. Interstate Ave. to starting point.

CONNECTING THE WALKS

The starting point of this walk makes for an easy connection with Walk 26: Columbia River Walk.

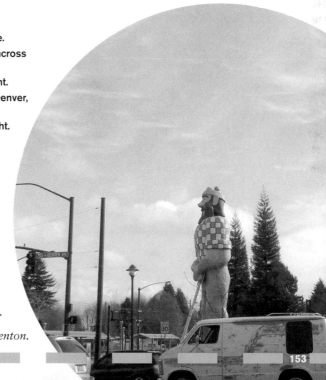

The Paul Bunyan statue keeps an eye on Kenton.

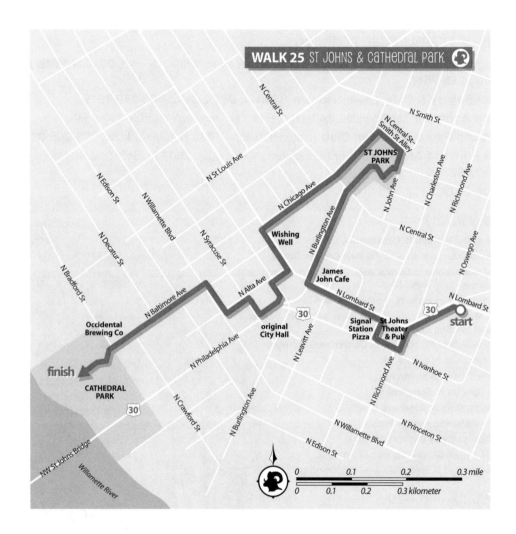

N Smith St

N Central St

N Central St-
Smith St Alley

ST JOHNS
PARK

N Charleston Ave

N Richmond Ave

N St Louis Ave

N Chicago Ave

N John Ave

N Central St

N Oswego Ave

N Edison St

N Willamette Blvd

N Syracuse St

N Burlington Ave

Wishing
Well

N Decatur St

James
John Cafe

N Lombard St

N Lombard St

N Bradford St

N Baltimore Ave

N Alta Ave

30

original
City Hall

N Leavitt Ave

30

Signal
Station
Pizza

St Johns
Theater
& Pub

Occidental
Brewing Co

start

N Philadelphia Ave

N Richmond Ave

N Ivanhoe St

finish

CATHEDRAL
PARK

30

N Crawford St

N Burlington Ave

N Willamette Blvd

N Princeton St

NW St Johns Bridge

Willamette River

N Edison St

| 0 | 0.1 | 0.2 | 0.3 mile |
| 0 | 0.1 | 0.2 | 0.3 kilometer |

25

ST. JOHNS AND CATHEDRAL PARK: SO FAR AWAY, SO CLOSE

BOUNDARIES: **N. Smith St., N. New York Ave., N. Ida Ave., Willamette River**
DISTANCE: **2 miles**
DIFFICULTY: **Moderate**
PARKING: **Free street parking, lot at Cathedral Park**
PUBLIC TRANSIT: **TriMet Bus 75 (N. Lombard St. and Oswego Ave.) or Buses 11 and 16 (N. Ivanhoe St. and Baltimore Ave.)**

Lots of Portlanders have close friends they claim they never see anymore because the friends bought houses in St. Johns and it's *soooo* far away. And there may be something to that: despite its many charms, this little neighborhood is not exactly handy. It's about 9 miles and a 15- to 20-minute drive from downtown Portland. But homes are still (for now) comparatively affordable here, and a few years back Portland's cool/bored-with-it-all crowd discovered that St. Johns has a huge amount of off-kilter charm (and a disproportionately high number of great bars for its size). It also has one of the area's most appealing parks and the prettiest bridge, hands-down. The saint in question, if you're curious, is James John, an early California import; he claimed a patch of land in 1843 and started platting the town.

● Start at the bus stop at N. Lombard St. and Oswego Ave. Walk along Lombard toward town. Bear left with N. Richmond St., then turn right on N. Ivanhoe St.

● At the corner of Richmond and Ivanhoe is the St. Johns Pub. Built in 1905 for the Lewis and Clark Expo, the pub was actually intended as a movie theater from the start, although it wasn't in St. Johns at the time. A church had it barged here on the Willamette River after the exposition; in fact, it served as a church more than once, and as an American Legion hall, before becoming a pub in 1989. It's now owned by the McMenamins, part of their mini-chain of microbrew theater pubs. The dome you see is not the original, but it's still very cute, and the inside has loads of charm. (Plus beer, pizza, and movies—you really can't go wrong.)

- Take N. Ivanhoe St. to N. Charleston Ave. and turn right. Check out Signal Station Pizza, an old Art Deco gas station converted into a pizzeria. Hang a left onto N. Lombard St.

- Continue along Lombard through what is essentially the main business strip of St. Johns. Stroll slowly and do a little window-shopping as you go. You'll also find a number of good spots for a bite; we're partial to the James John Cafe for brunch or breakfast, but you should explore.

- At N. Burlington Ave., turn right. Cross N. Central St. and head into St. Johns Park. Make a loop around the park, then cross back over Central and onto N. Chicago Ave. When you get to N. Lombard St., turn left. A block farther is The Wishing Well, a great dive bar in an excellent building, with a cool sign to boot.

- Turn right on N. Alta Ave., then left on N. Ivanhoe St. At N. Philadelphia Ave. turn right. The redbrick building across the street was originally City Hall, built in 1905. It's now occupied by a training division of the Portland Police.

- At N. Syracuse St. take a right to get back onto N. Alta Ave., onto which you'll turn left and walk a block before turning right on N. Willamette Blvd., then left on N. Baltimore Ave. to head down a steep hill toward the river.

- Just past N. Decatur St. stands a big orange industrial-looking building. In its courtyard you'll find, among a handful of other businesses, Occidental Brewing Co., a scrappy little microbrewery with excellent beers and a teeny-tiny bar in the corner of its factory space. Well worth stopping in; you can also get a growler of beer to take with you.

- Beyond the brewery, cross the railroad tracks and go straight to enter Cathedral Park. This is one of the nicest parks in Portland, only partly because of its awesome view of the St. Johns Bridge, whose 40-story-tall Gothic cathedral spires and slender silhouette look good from pretty much any angle. The St. Johns Bridge was built in 1931 by David B. Steinman, who built an awful lot of bridges in his time but claimed this one as his favorite. As for the park, it was recognized as a good hangout early on: Lewis and Clark apparently stopped here, camping overnight, in 1806. It was also the landing point for the ferry between St. Johns and Linnton, across the river. But it didn't officially become a park until 1980. These days it's the site of an annual jazz festival, as well as the new venue for the very Portland phenomenon called Trek in the Park. (It's a crew of local theater people reproducing *Star Trek* episodes live on an outdoor stage all summer— it's awesome and massively popular. Go to atomic-arts.org for more info.)

● It's a fairly steep climb back up the hill to the starting point. Walk up N. Ivanhoe St. until you reach N. Lombard St., where you can either catch Bus 44 or turn right and walk back to N. Oswego Ave., where we began.

POINTS OF INTEREST (START TO FINISH)

St. Johns Theater & Pub mcmenamins.com/stjohns, 8203 N. Ivanhoe St., 503-283-8520

Signal Station Pizza signalstationpizza.com, 8302 N. Lombard St., 503-286-2257

James John Cafe jamesjohncafe.com, 8527 N. Lombard St., 503-285-4930

Wishing Well 8800 N. Lombard St., 503-286-4434

Occidental Brewing Co. occidentalbrewing.com, 6635 N. Baltimore Ave., 503-719-7102

ROUTE SUMMARY

1. Start at the corner of N. Lombard St. and Oswego Ave.
2. From Lombard, bear left at N. Richmond St.
3. Turn right on N. Ivanhoe St.
4. Turn right on N. Charleston Ave.
5. Turn left on N. Lombard St.
6. Turn right at N. Burlington Ave.
7. Cross N. Central St. to St. Johns Park.
8. Exit the park, recrossing N. Central onto N. Chicago Ave.
9. Turn left on N. Lombard St.
10. Turn right on N. Alta Ave.
11. Turn left on N. Ivanhoe St.
12. Turn right on N. Philadelphia Ave.
13. Turn right on N. Syracuse St.
14. Turn left on N. Alta Ave.
15. Turn right on N. Willamette Blvd.
16. Turn left on N. Baltimore Ave.
17. Cross the train tracks to reach Cathedral Park.
18. Retrace your steps up to N. Lombard St. to return to starting point.

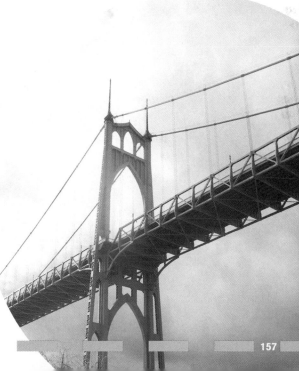

The St. Johns Bridge
(Photo courtesy of Paul Gerald)

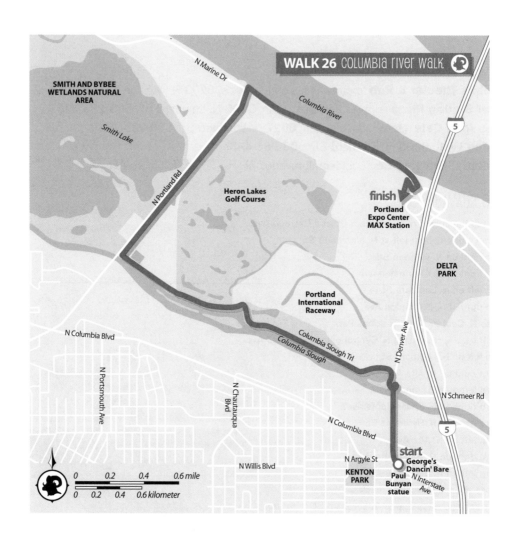

SMITH AND BYBEE
WETLANDS NATURAL
AREA

Smith Lake

N Marine Dr

Columbia River

N Portland Rd

Heron Lakes
Golf Course

finish

Portland
Expo Center
MAX Station

DELTA
PARK

Portland
International
Raceway

N Columbia Blvd

N Portsmouth Ave

Columbia Slough Trl
Columbia Slough

N Chautauqua
Blvd

N Denver Ave

N Schmeer Rd

N Columbia Blvd

N Willis Blvd

N Argyle St

KENTON
PARK

Paul
Bunyan
statue

start
George's
Dancin' Bare

N Interstate
Ave

0   0.2   0.4   0.6 mile
0   0.2   0.4   0.6 kilometer

26

COLUMBIA RIVER WALK: DESOLATION ROW

BOUNDARIES: **N. Marine Dr., N. Portland Rd., Columbia Slough, I-5**
DISTANCE: **5 miles**
DIFFICULTY: **Easy**
PARKING: **Free street parking**
PUBLIC TRANSIT: **TriMet Interstate MAX Yellow Line (Kenton/N. Denver Ave., Expo Center Stations)**

This is a great-wide-open, middle-of-nowhere, get-out-and-stretch-your-legs walk. Though it passes by several heavy-industry areas, with all the accompanying toxic leftovers, it also incorporates some of the more interesting natural features of the Portland region and the site of a historic residential development that was needlessly destroyed in a flood. In short, this walk provides plenty of opportunity to meditate on things that have vanished without a trace, as well as the things we leave behind that can never be completely erased. There's not a lot in the way of refreshments or entertainment out here, so bring whatever supplies you might need, and prepare to cover a bit of ground.

● Start at the Kenton/N. Denver Ave. MAX Station. Take a moment to marvel at the statue of Paul Bunyan on the far side of the MAX tracks. (For more about him, see Walk 24: Historic Kenton.) Staying on the north side of the tracks, take the sidewalk past George's Dancin' Bare—bet you can't guess what that is—and cross N. Argyle St. Cross the MAX tracks and continue onto the pedestrian strip along the N. Denver Ave. overpass.

● Follow N. Denver across the Columbia Slough, then duck to the right onto a corkscrew walkway leading down to N. Schmeer Rd. This loops beneath Denver Ave.; carefully cross Schmeer and veer left to join the Columbia Slough Trail.

● To your right is, among other things, the Portland International Raceway, where the Oregon Motorcycle Road Racing Association (omrra.com) holds competitive events throughout the summer; there are also weekly drag races and motocross competitions, trade shows, "drifting" demos, and all manner of gearhead entertainment. If there's a race on when you're in the area, it's well worth going to see. (Or better yet, volunteer as a corner worker, where you get free admission, free lunch, and the best view of the races. Details about volunteering are on OMRRA's website—anybody can do it; all it takes is showing up the morning of the event.)

● The body of water you're walking alongside, the Columbia Slough, is part of a complicated wetlands system making up a 60-mile watershed in North Portland. The slough parallels the Columbia River for 18 miles until its confluence with the Willamette. Over the years, the surrounding industry (not to mention general drainage from Portland) has left the slough polluted, but it's still used as a recreational zone (for kayaking, hiking, etc.) and continues to serve its original function as part of the city's flood-control system.

● Follow the Columbia Slough Trail until you see the railroad bridge at N. Portland Rd. Turn right onto the walking path alongside N. Portland and follow it through a wild, remote industrial zone. On your left is Smith Lake, part of the Smith and Bybee Wetlands Natural Area, the largest protected wetlands area within a city in the United States. On your right are Heron Lakes Golf Course and the former site of Vanport City.

During the 1940s, Vanport was the largest wartime housing development in the country. Defense workers rushing to Portland, mostly in shipbuilding, needed a place to live, so in 1942 a 650-acre parcel of the Columbia River floodplain was turned into a massive housing project. More than 9,000 apartments were built on the swampy land; with more than 40,000 residents at its peak, Vanport was the second-largest city in Oregon. It was also racially segregated and generally discontent; the Housing Authority of Portland at the time called it "troublesome" and "blighted."

After the war ended, most of the people who stayed on in Vanport were African Americans. On Memorial Day in 1948, the Columbia River overflowed its floodplain. Residents of Vanport had all of 35 minutes to escape. The hastily built wooden apartments washed away in moments; within hours, nothing was left. At least 15 people died. Rumors lingered that authorities had purposely neglected to warn Vanport residents until the last minute. In any case, those who'd been flooded out of their homes suddenly had nowhere to live; many of them settled in North and Northeast Portland, establishing what was to become the heart of Portland's black community.

● At the river, cross N. Marine Dr. and turn right. (The land you see across the water is Hayden Island, home to the Jantzen Beach shopping area and, to the west, a lot of undeveloped land that may soon be annexed to Portland. The debate over what to do with the west side of Hayden Island has been referred to in local press as a "land grab," and it seems an ugly fight may be in store.) You are now walking parallel to the Oregon section of the Columbia River (the Washington state line is on the other side of Hayden Island). Follow the trail along the water's edge until it curves back in toward N. Marine Dr. (also known as N. Swift Hwy. and OR 120).

- At the stoplight where N. Marine Dr. meets NE Martin Luther King Jr. Blvd., cross Marine Dr., then turn right (heading back in the direction you came from) about 100 meters until you see on your left the walkway to the Portland Expo Center MAX Station. Follow this curved path to the station, where the Yellow Line will take you back into town.

POINTS OF INTEREST (START TO FINISH)

George's Dancin' Bare georgesdancinbare.com, 8440 N. Interstate Ave., 503-285-9073

Portland International Raceway portlandraceway.com, 1940 N. Victory Blvd.

Smith and Bybee Wetlands Natural Area 5300 N. Marine Dr.

ROUTE SUMMARY

1. Start at the Kenton/N. Denver Ave. MAX Station.

2. Cross N. Argyle St.

3. Cross the MAX tracks and turn right onto N. Denver Ave.

4. Turn right to reach N. Schmeer Rd.

5. Veer left onto the Columbia Slough Trail.

6. Turn right onto the footpath at N. Portland Rd.

7. Cross N. Marine Dr. and turn right.

8. At the stoplight, cross N. Marine Dr. and turn right.

9. Turn left onto the MAX station walkway.

CONNECTING THE WALKS

The starting point of this walk makes for an easy connection with Walk 24: Historic Kenton.

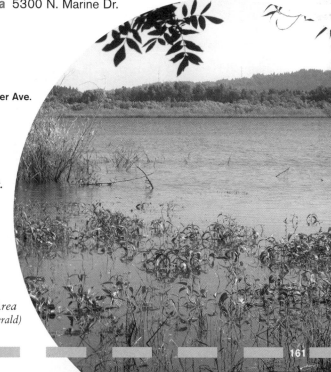

Smith and Bybee Wetlands Natural Area
(Photo courtesy of Paul Gerald)

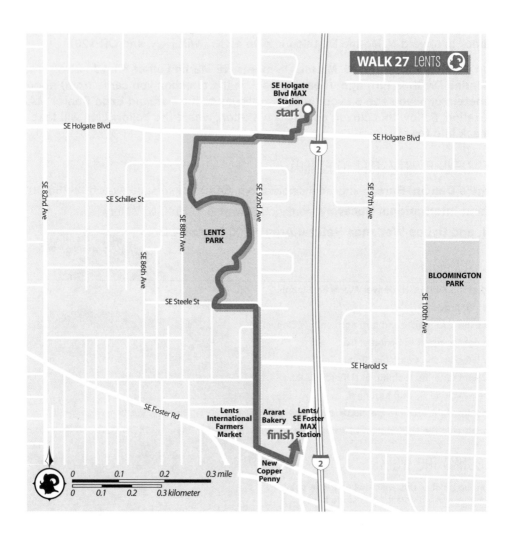

SE Holgate
Blvd MAX
Station
start

SE Holgate Blvd

SE Holgate Blvd

2

SE 82nd Ave

SE Schiller St

SE 92nd Ave

SE 97th Ave

SE 88th Ave

LENTS
PARK

BLOOMINGTON
PARK

SE 86th Ave

SE 100th Ave

SE Steele St

SE Harold St

SE Foster Rd

Lents
International
Farmers
Market

Ararat
Bakery

Lents/
SE Foster
MAX
Station

finish

New
Copper
Penny

2

0   0.1   0.2   0.3 mile
0   0.1   0.2   0.3 kilometer

27

LENTS: a TOWN CUT IN TWO

BOUNDARIES: SE 92nd Ave., SE Holgate Blvd., SE 72nd Ave., SE Woodstock Blvd.
DISTANCE: 1.5 miles
DIFFICULTY: Easy
PARKING: Free street parking
PUBLIC TRANSIT: MAX Green Line (SE Holgate Blvd. and Lents/SE Foster Stations); you could also get here via the I-205 Multi-Use Path

The actual neighborhood of Lents—named after Oliver Perry Lent, a pioneer who ran a 190-acre farm in the area in 1866—is fairly large (nearly 4 square miles), but its downtown core is barely there. With all the boarded-up shopfronts and papered-over windows, it has an almost ghost-town appeal. This is mainly because Lents got the short end of the transit stick back when Portland was trying to figure out where the I-205 freeway should go. (It had been planned for 39th Avenue, but folks in the more powerful and moneyed Laurelhurst neighborhood wouldn't have it.) By running the freeway along Southeast 95th Avenue, city leaders basically cut Lents in half, leaving it more a traffic hub than anything else. Still, it's the center of one of the most diverse parts of Portland, with a higher number of Latino, Asian, and Russian immigrants than most other parts of town. Recently it has been named an Urban Renewal Area, which allows the city to use property-tax funds for improvement projects. And the weekly farmers' market here draws folks from much closer in, thanks to its ethnically diverse makeup and resulting tendency to have things you can't find at other markets. Things might be looking up for Lents . . . eventually.

● Start the walk at the SE Holgate Blvd. MAX Station, on the Green Line. From the station, cross Holgate and head right (east) until you reach SE 92nd Ave., where you'll enter Lents Park.

The park (like the neighborhood) is named for stonemason Oliver Lent, who had a land claim here in the 1850s. (It was his son who laid out the town plan in the 1890s; Portland annexed it in 1912.) Locals have been gathering up land to use as park space since the 1940s, and the city established an official plan for its layout in 1953. The park includes a good-sized stadium ringed with trees, plus a couple of smaller softball fields, two soccer fields, tennis courts, and footpaths linking them all. At the southern end, picnic tables are arranged beneath beautiful old-growth trees.

● Wander the length of Lents Park along the footpaths until you reach its southern boundary, at SE Steele St.; turn left to get back to SE 92nd Ave. At 92nd, turn right and walk several blocks toward Lents's town center, such as it is.

● At the corner of SE 92nd Ave. and Ramona St. you'll find the Ararat Bakery, which is not only a bakery but also a restaurant (serving fantastic Eastern European–style home cooking) and sometimes an after-hours lounge, depending on the day and the hour. There's also a shop section where you can pick up imported goodies as well as take-home versions of the baked goods.

● Diagonally across SE 92nd Ave. is the site of the Lents International Farmers Market (Sundays 11 a.m.–4 p.m., June–October), a relatively new market with a cosmopolitan vibe so pronounced that the posters and website that advertise it are rendered in five languages. The scope of its offerings has started to draw shoppers from far-off neighborhoods who are eager to try something new or hunting down a hard-to-find specialty. Compared with other Portland markets, it's on the small side, but it has a distinctive community-based feel that can't be missed.

● A few blocks farther up, past a Mexican restaurant, a dodgy-looking bar, and a sweet little coffee shop, you'll reach a stoplight and be faced with the New Copper Penny. It looks totally uninspiring from this angle. If you take a left up SE Foster Rd. and walk to the front entrance (you can't miss the huge neon penny), it looks a bit less dire (at night anyway) but is instead confusing: inside it's a gigantic nightclub–steakhouse–sports-bar combo with a large and well-equipped children's play area in one corner. Overall it has the feel of a relic, though from what era we can't quite say. But if you have kids with you and you'd like to park them somewhere while you enjoy a steak and some booze and maybe a UFC fight on TV, you're in luck.

● Cross back over to the other side of SE Foster Rd. and take the walkway left up to the Lents/SE Foster MAX Station, where you can catch the Green Line back into town.

POINTS OF INTEREST (START TO FINISH)

Ararat Bakery 5716 SE 92nd Ave., 503-235-5526

Lents International Farmers Market lentsfarmersmarket.org, SE 92nd Ave. and Foster Rd.

New Copper Penny 5932 SE 92nd Ave., 503-777-1415

ROUTE SUMMARY

1. Start at the **SE Holgate Blvd. MAX Station.**
2. Turn right onto **SE Holgate Blvd.**
3. Enter Lents Park at **SE 92nd Ave. and Holgate.**
4. Walk to south side of park.
5. Turn left on **SE Steele St.**
6. Turn right on **SE 92nd Ave.**
7. Turn left on **SE Foster Rd.**
8. Turn left to reach the **Lents/SE Foster MAX Station.**

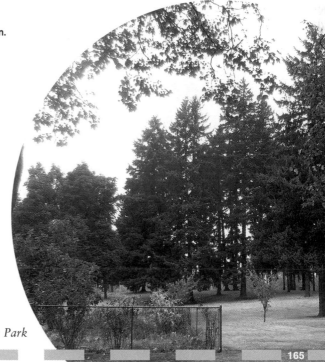

Community garden at Lents Park

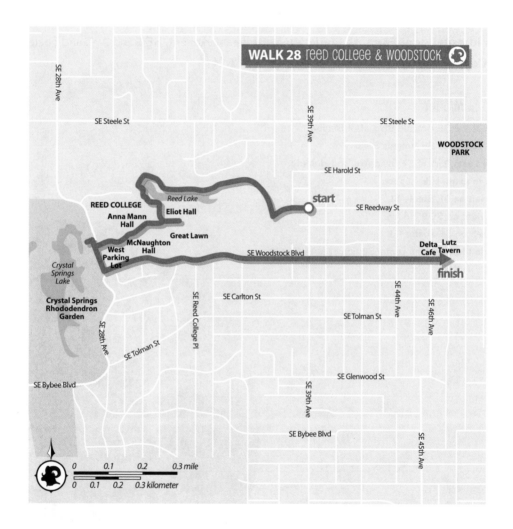

SE 28th Ave

SE 39th Ave

SE Steele St

SE Steele St

WOODSTOCK PARK

SE Harold St

REED COLLEGE

Reed Lake

start

SE Reedway St

Anna Mann Hall

Eliot Hall

Great Lawn

West Parking Lot

McNaughton Hall

Crystal Springs Lake

SE Woodstock Blvd

Delta Cafe

Lutz Tavern

finish

Crystal Springs Rhododendron Garden

SE 28th Ave

SE Reed College Pl

SE Carlton St

SE 44th Ave

SE 46th Ave

SE Tolman St

SE Tolman St

SE Glenwood St

SE 39th Ave

SE 45th Ave

SE Bybee Blvd

SE Bybee Blvd

0   0.1   0.2   0.3 mile

0   0.1   0.2   0.3 kilometer

28 reed college and woodstock: communism, atheism, free love

BOUNDARIES: **SE Woodstock Blvd., SE 28th Ave., SE 47th Ave., SE Steele St.**
DISTANCE: **2.5 miles (not including optional Crystal Springs Rhododendron Garden detour)**
DIFFICULTY: **Easy**
PARKING: **On street, small lot on campus**
PUBLIC TRANSIT: **TriMet Bus 75 (SE Cesar Chavez Blvd. and Harold or Knight St.) or Bus 19 (SE Woodstock Blvd. and 46th Ave.)**

Reed College occupies a beautiful campus surrounded by an equally attractive residential neighborhood. Founded in 1908 and named for Oregon pioneers Simeon and Amanda Reed, the school is uniquely and legendarily progressive. (Its unofficial motto is "Communism, Atheism, Free Love.") Apple founder Steve Jobs famously dropped out—he often credited a calligraphy class he took at Reed with helping him figure out computer fonts and backgrounds. Other notable Reedies include journalist Barbara Ehrenreich, poet Gary Snyder, and (briefly) musician Ry Cooder. The students here work their tails off (Reed produces disproportionately high numbers of Rhodes Scholars and PhDs and is notorious for academic rigor), but anyone can enjoy strolling the grounds without so much as setting foot in a library. Add in a side trip through Crystal Springs Rhododendron Garden before you head up the hill into the heart of the charming Woodstock neighborhood.

● Start at SE 39th Ave. and Reedway St. Walk down the hill on Reedway to SE 38th Ave. and find the little dirt trail that leads down into the woods. This path winds through Reed Canyon, alongside Crystal Springs Creek and around Reed Lake. The canyon is a 28-acre watershed that essentially bisects the Reed College campus. It's home to a range of interesting plants and wild animals (and no, we don't mean the students—more like garter snakes and birds). Where the trail forks, bear right, which will lead you meanderingly around the north side of Reed Lake. Eventually you'll come to a gray concrete-and-steel bridge; don't cross it, but pass underneath it and continue along the trail.

● The trail ends when it meets a gravel road. Turn left here and walk through a small parking lot, then up the stairs. You'll be facing Cerf Auditorium, built in 1936 and named for a Reed lit professor. Keeping the auditorium to your left, walk up the hill along the cement path. Stay on the path as it sweeps left, across the top of the auditorium, then sneaks behind a large gray building. Keep your eye on the windows to your right as you walk by, and you'll catch a glimpse of a mural of comic-book characters, including *Transmetropolitan*'s Spider Jerusalem: this is the entrance to the totally awesome Reed comics library, called the MLLL (mlll.org—the website has a pretty useful comic-book-recommendation engine).

● Follow the cement path around the corner of the building, uphill, and to the right. You'll emerge onto the lawn behind the Student Union; to your left is Eliot Hall. Walk straight ahead onto the Great Lawn, a vast, open, tree-dotted area that's ideal for a picnic, reading, napping, maybe some croquet, or just appreciating the lovely campus, whose plan was loosely modeled on St. John's College at Oxford.

Eliot Hall—more or less the architectural centerpiece of the campus—was built in 1912, in the same Tudor Gothic style that defines the other impressive building you see from the lawn, Old Dorm Block. Look for the Reed College seal over the southwest corner of Eliot Hall; it incorporates roses as well as fleurs-de-lis from Washington University in St. Louis, where Thomas Lamb Eliot went to school. There are 13 stars borrowed from the family crest of John Adams, a relation of Amanda Reed's. The griffin on the seal is Reed's unofficial mascot—it has a lion's body with an eagle's head and is associated with protection and wisdom. Eliot himself was that rare creature, a powerful clergyman in the Pacific Northwest. He came to Portland in 1867 to serve as minister at the large new Unitarian Church. He worked for a number of progressive causes, including education, child welfare, and women's suffrage, and he served on the Reed College board of trustees for 20 years. Adding to his brainy bona fides, he was the uncle of literary giant T. S. Eliot.

Eliot Hall is also where the Reed experience culminates, at least academically: seniors have to write a thesis in order to graduate, and it's a rigorous undertaking. So each year at the end of the semester, all the seniors who managed to complete it make two extra copies of their thesis (having turned in the real one already) and embark on the Thesis Parade, in which a ragtag marching band leads the seniors into

Eliot Hall and up to the registrar's office, where one by one they each plunk down their thesis, symbolically and with much fanfare handing it in. (The second extra copy is then ceremoniously burned in a bonfire right in front of the library.) Then everyone gets drunk and high in the rain.

● From the Great Lawn, in front of Eliot Hall and Old Dorm Block, wander downhill (west) between Anna Mann (the pretty gray dorm to your right) and McNaughton (a newer, less pretty dorm) toward the campus's West Parking Lot. (This slope is usually the location of the naked waterslide during Reed's annual Renn Fayre, FYI.) Carefully cross the street (SE 28th Ave.) to the entrance of Crystal Springs Rhododendron Garden.

If time allows, Crystal Springs makes for a very pleasant detour. Once upon a time, the land now occupied by the garden was Crystal Springs Farm, owned by William Ladd, of Ladd's Addition and Laurelhurst Park fame (see Back Story: William S. Ladd, page 82). Before it became a botanical garden, it was used as an outdoor theater (Reedies apparently used to call it "Shakespeare Island"). The land found its true calling in the 1950s, as a botanical test garden. Over the years it has gradually been developed, shaped, and landscaped (partly using rocks from Mt. Hood) and now contains some 2,500 azaleas, rhododendrons, and other plants. Mostly it's just a really pretty place to wander around, look at some fountains, see masses of surrealistically colorful flowers in bloom, and so forth.

● Leaving the garden, take a right on SE 28th Ave. and then a left onto SE Woodstock Blvd. Follow Woodstock up the hill, alongside a residential area of upscale homes and quiet, tree-lined side streets. Cross SE 39th Ave. at the stoplight at the hill's summit, and continue along Woodstock Blvd. (On your right as you cross 39th Ave., you'll see a dilapidated yellowy-beige house on the corner—this is a long-established Reed party house called the Dustbin, where many good times have been forgotten.)

● At SE 43rd Ave., look left to peek at the Woodstock Community Center. It's housed in a restored firehouse from 1928 and holds classes for kids and adults alike, in everything from tae kwon do to fingerpainting.

● Lots of eating and drinking establishments line this stretch of Woodstock, but one of the friendlier and livelier options is the Delta Cafe, just past SE 46th Ave., where you can get Southern home cooking and a 40-ounce bottle of Pabst Blue Ribbon served in a bucket of ice like Champagne.

● Before or after visiting the Delta, pop in at the Lutz Tavern, a beloved Reed student hangout next door. Recent changes in ownership have left it looking like a bar in search of an identity, but it has a long history and an easygoing vibe.

● From here, retrace your steps back down the hill to SE 39th Ave., turn right, and reach the starting point, or catch a bus at Woodstock Blvd. and 46th Ave. toward downtown.

POINTS OF INTEREST (START TO FINISH)

Reed College reed.edu

Crystal Springs Rhododendron Garden rhodies.org, SE 28th Ave. and Woodstock Blvd., 503-771-8386

Woodstock Community Center 5905 SE 43rd Ave., 503-823-3633

Delta Cafe deltacafepdx.com, 4607 SE Woodstock Blvd., 503-771-3101

Lutz Tavern 4639 SE Woodstock Blvd., 503-774-0353

ROUTE SUMMARY

1. Start at SE 39th Ave. and Reedway St.
2. Walk downhill 1 block on Reedway to the trail entrance.
3. At the fork in the trail, bear right.
4. At the gravel road, turn left.
5. Cross the parking lot and go up the stairs.
6. Take the cement path to the top of Cerf Auditorium.
7. At the top of Cerf, turn left.
8. Follow path to the right onto the lawn.
9. Turn right (west) at the Great Lawn.
10. Cross SE 28th Ave. to Crystal Springs Rhododendron Garden.
11. Exiting the garden, turn right on SE 28th Ave.
12. Turn left at the stop sign, up SE Woodstock Blvd.
13. Follow SE Woodstock Blvd. up the hill to end of route.

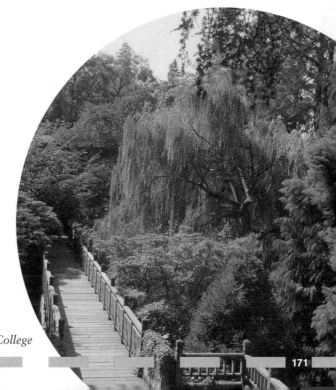

Crystal Springs Rhododendron Garden, near Reed College

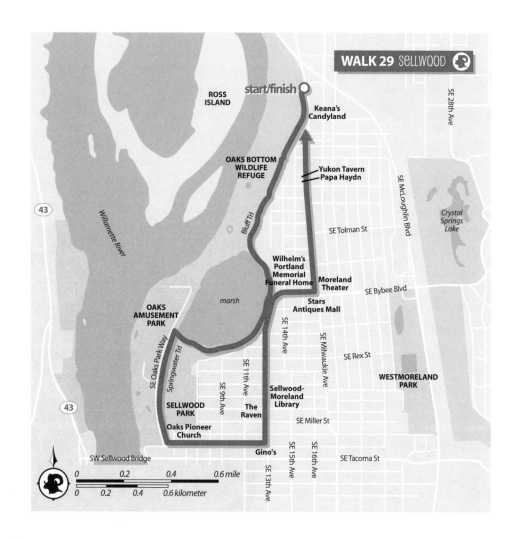

ROSS
ISLAND

start/finish

Keana's
Candyland

OAKS BOTTOM
WILDLIFE
REFUGE

Yukon Tavern
Papa Haydn

SE 28th Ave

Crystal
Springs
Lake

SE McLoughlin Blvd

Willamette River

43

Bluff Trl

SE Tolman St

Wilhelm's
Portland
Memorial
Funeral Home

Moreland
Theater

SE Bybee Blvd

OAKS
AMUSEMENT
PARK

marsh

Stars
Antiques Mall

SE 14th Ave

SE Milwaukie Ave

SE Rex St

WESTMORELAND
PARK

SE Oaks Park Way

Springwater Trl

SE 9th Ave

SE 11th Ave

Sellwood-
Moreland
Library

43

SELLWOOD
PARK

The Raven

SE Miller St

Oaks Pioneer
Church

Gino's

SE 13th Ave

SE 15th Ave

SE 16th Ave

SE Tacoma St

SW Sellwood Bridge

| 0 | 0.2 | 0.4 | 0.6 mile |
| 0 | 0.2 | 0.4 | 0.6 kilometer |

29 seLLWOOD: ANTIQUE JUNGLE

BOUNDARIES: **SE Milwaukie Ave., SE Tacoma St., and the Willamette River**
DISTANCE: **4 miles**
DIFFICULTY: **Easy–moderate**
PARKING: **Small free lot at start/finish; nearby street parking also available**
PUBLIC TRANSIT: **TriMet Bus 19 (numerous stops along SE Milwaukie Ave.)**

Annexed by Portland in 1893, Sellwood for many years was its own incorporated town, and it still has the independent, off-the-main-drag feel of "elsewhere." The neighborhood is known primarily for Antique Row, the nickname for SE 13th Avenue, although these days many of the antiques stores along the street have been replaced by restaurants and coffee shops. Sellwood's other claim to fame is Oaks Amusement Park, a charmingly low-key family-fun spot with year-round roller skating, and the abutting Oaks Bottom Wildlife Refuge, a great place for bird-watching. The trail through the refuge is part of the Springwater Corridor trail network, which in turn is part of the metro area's 40-Mile Loop trail system. (The Springwater Trail currently runs 21 miles from industrial Southeast Portland to the town of Boring; plans call for eventually connecting it to the Pacific Crest Trail.) The narrow, 85-year-old Sellwood Bridge is Portland's southernmost; it was built on a budget and is about to undergo an elaborate makeover, partly to improve its earthquake-readiness.

● Start at the small parking lot for Oaks Bottom Wildlife Refuge, where SE Milwaukie Ave. meets Mitchell St., just north of Sellwood proper. The refuge includes about 160 acres of woodlands and wetlands and serves as home or landing strip to more than a hundred bird species. A paved footpath descends into the woodlands between Sellwood and the river. After about 500 meters, the pavement swoops right, toward the river and the Springwater Trail—instead, you'll take the Bluff Trail, a narrower dirt path that continues straight.

● About 800 meters farther along, look uphill to your left to see the backside of Wilhelm's Portland Memorial Funeral Home, which has been cheerily brightened up with paintings of birds on the lake (but remains, somehow, just a little creepy). The opposite side of the trail here is a dense marshland that feels quite far from the bustling neighborhood just over the ridge.

- After circling the marsh, the Bluff Trail runs smack into the Springwater Trail at Oaks Amusement Park. Here you'll find a roller-skating rink, carnival rides, go-karts, bumper cars, and a well-worn collection of midway entertainments. If you stop in, don't miss the hand-carved wooden carousel from 1912.

- Continue south along the Springwater Trail until you reach the tiny Oaks Pioneer Church, at SE Spokane St. Born in 1851 as the St. Johns Episcopal Church in Milwaukie (south of Sellwood), the little white building moved twice before settling here. After 10 years it was scooted closer to SE Main St. in Milwaukie. Then, in 1883, the church got a remodel, adding its current stained-glass windows and steeple. In the 1950s it moved again, to SE Jefferson St. in Milwaukie, where it served as a Sunday-school annex to a larger church building and suffered the indignity of having linoleum floors installed. But its big adventure came in the 1960s, when it was spared from demolition and instead loaded onto a barge and shipped up the Willamette River to its current home, where (linoleum-free) it's a popular spot for weddings and funerals.

- Walk up the hill along SE Spokane St. until you reach SE 13th Ave. Gino's, on the corner, is a beautiful old family-style Italian restaurant with a lovely bar, if you're in need of sustenance. Otherwise, turn left and continue along 13th Ave. into the heart of Sellwood.

- SE 13th Ave. is Sellwood's "Antique Row," lined with antiques shops (though these days they battle for space with new restaurants and coffee shops). There's a pretty good range of inventory, from high-end and rare items to cardboard boxes full of broken Legos and one-legged baby dolls. A longstanding favorite is The Raven, between SE Miller and Lexington Sts., with appealingly curmudgeonly staff and an emphasis on old military and maritime gear.

- A block farther, at SE Bidwell St., is the Sellwood-Moreland branch of the Multnomah County Library. Started in 1905 as the Sellwood Reading Room with 100 books, in a small building on Nehalem St., the library moved into this successful experiment in mixed-use architecture in 2002. The building also contains commercial space and 16 condominiums.

- Continue along SE 13th Ave. until it rounds a bend and, at SE 14th Ave., becomes SE Bybee Blvd. Here you can also peek into the pretty grounds of the somewhat-less-creepy Memorial Funeral Home. Follow SE Bybee Blvd. until it meets SE Milwaukie Ave. (at which point those so inclined may want to duck half a block right for another antiques powerhouse, Stars Antiques Mall). Turn left on Milwaukie Ave. to walk through the tiny heart of Sellwood.

- One of Portland's handful of historic single-screen movie houses, the Moreland Theater (1926), is on the right. Look for the Johnson Jewelers clock, a familiar landmark, out front.

- Continuing along SE Milwaukie Ave., you'll find plenty of chances for refreshment, but wait until you reach the yin–yang duo that is Papa Haydn and the Yukon Tavern. The former is a delightfully upscale restaurant known for its desserts, with a lovely outdoor garden in the warmer months; the Yukon, on the other hand, is an excellent dive with faded red-velvet walls, cheap drinks, and ancient regulars glued to their disintegrating barstools. You really can't lose either way.

- The final stretch of SE Milwaukie Ave. leading back to the Oaks Bottom parking lot features one of Sellwood's oddest mysteries: Keana's Candyland, an inexplicably unsettling gingerbread house encrusted with plastic candy canes, outsize lollipops, Christmas lights, and hand-drawn signs that beckon you in, Hansel and Gretel–like, past the white picket fence. It's allegedly just a bakery and candy shop, but those who fear unicorns and magic are advised to approach with caution.

- Continue another 100 meters or so along SE Milwaukie Ave. to reach the Oaks Bottom parking lot.

POINTS OF INTEREST (START TO FINISH)

Oaks Bottom Wildlife Refuge tinyurl.com/oaksbottom, SE Milwaukie Ave. and Mitchell St.

Wilhelm's Portland Memorial Funeral Home 6705 SE 14th Ave.

Oaks Amusement Park oakspark.com, 7805 SE Oaks Park Way, 503-233-5777

Oaks Pioneer Church oakspioneerchurch.org, 455 SE Spokane St.

Gino's ginossellwood.com, 8051 SE 13th Ave., 503-233-4613

The Raven ravenantiques.com, 7927 SE 13th Ave., 503-233-8075

Sellwood-Moreland Library multcolib.org, 7860 SE 13th Ave., 503-988-5398

Stars Antiques Mall starsantique.com, 7027 SE Milwaukie Ave., 503-239-0346

Moreland Theater morelandtheater.com, 6712 SE Milwaukie Ave., 503-236-5257

Papa Haydn papahaydn.com, 5829 SE Milwaukie Ave., 503-232-9440

Yukon Tavern 5819 SE Milwaukie Ave., 503-235-6352

Keana's Candyland keanascandyland.net, 5314 SE Milwaukie Ave., 503-719-5131

route summary

1. Start at the Oaks Bottom parking lot at SE Milwaukie Ave. and Mitchell St.
2. Follow the paved trail downhill into the woods.
3. Continue straight along the Bluff Trail.
4. Merge onto the Springwater Trail.
5. Turn left on SE Spokane St.
6. Turn left on SE 13th Ave.
7. Turn left at SE Milwaukie Ave. and follow it to starting point.

Connecting the Walks

The Springwater Corridor Trail continues north into Portland proper, near the Oregon Museum of Science and Industry (OMSI), where you can link with Walk 12: Industrial Southeast.

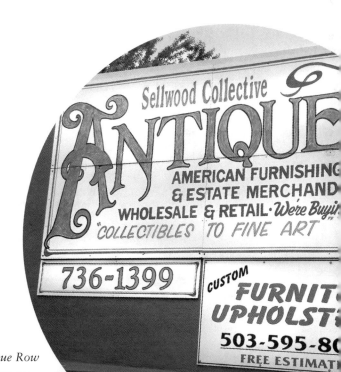

A mural on Sellwood's Antique Row

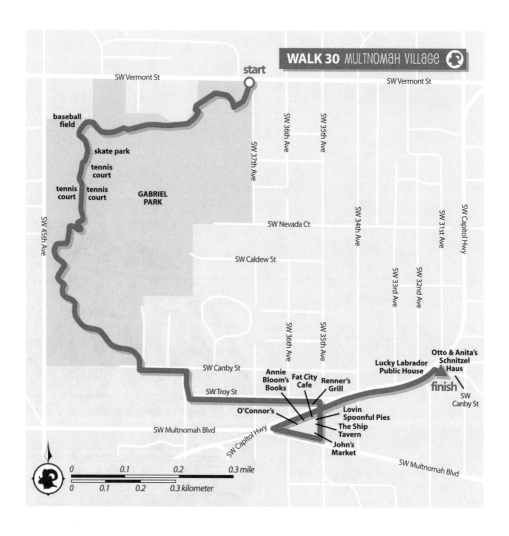

start

SW Vermont St

SW Vermont St

baseball
field

skate park

tennis
court

tennis
court

tennis
court

GABRIEL
PARK

SW 45th Ave

SW 37th Ave

SW 36th Ave

SW 35th Ave

SW 34th Ave

SW 33rd Ave

SW 32nd Ave

SW 31st Ave

SW Capitol Hwy

SW Nevada Ct

SW Caldew St

SW Canby St

SW Troy St

SW Multnomah Blvd

SW Capitol Hwy

SW 36th Ave

SW 35th Ave

Annie
Bloom's
Books

Fat City
Cafe

Renner's
Grill

O'Connor's

Lovin
Spoonful Pies

The Ship
Tavern

John's
Market

Lucky Labrador
Public House

Otto & Anita's
Schnitzel
Haus

finish

SW
Canby St

SW Multnomah Blvd

0   0.1   0.2   0.3 mile

0   0.1   0.2   0.3 kilometer

30 MULTNOMAH VILLAGE: SMALL BUT FILLING

BOUNDARIES: **SW Vermont St., SW 45th Ave., SW Multnomah Blvd., SW 30th Ave.**
DISTANCE: **1.75 miles**
DIFFICULTY: **Easy**
PARKING: **Free street parking, lots at Gabriel Park**
PUBLIC TRANSIT: **TriMet Buses 1 and 45 (SW Vermont St. and 37th Ave.) or Bus 44
     (SW Capitol Hwy. and 33rd Ave.)**

Built around an Oregon Electric Railway depot and annexed by Portland in 1950, Multnomah Village is a cute, pocket-size neighborhood just out of the way enough to be neglected by many Portlanders. It feels like a trek from the city center, but in fact it's only about 5 miles from downtown and easily accessible by bus. The downtown core is a very compact area with a surprising variety of shops, bars, and cafes. And the surrounding areas are lovely— thick with trees and rich in green spaces, including nearby Gabriel Park, where our walk begins. Though Multnomah Village is an easy drive from Portland proper, we recommend using public transportation if you can, particularly if you plan to take advantage of the neighborhood's disproportionately high number of excellent dive bars. This is a point-to-point walk with bus stops at either end, so playing it safe should be easy.

● Start the walk at the northeast corner of Gabriel Park—there's a bus stop here and another a few blocks east. The path forks a few feet from the entrance; take the right-hand branch and follow its meandering path across to the west side of the park. Gabriel Park is a 90-acre playground with something for just about everyone. Paved and dirt trails wind all across the park, and you'll also find the usual picnic areas, ball fields, tennis courts, basketball courts, and dog parks. There's also a state-of-the-art play area for the little kids, and a skate park, built in 2008, for the slightly bigger kids. Along with a community garden, there's also a demonstration orchard. The park is named after a farmer who once owned this land (back in the 1890s), a Swiss immigrant named Ulrich Gabriel.

● At the baseball field, take the left-hand fork to pass the skate park. Follow the path between two tennis courts and continue straight as it heads into a more thickly forested area. This section of path winds through the woods for a while; you'll come out near the baseball diamond. Pass this and continue to a small parking lot, at the southeast corner of the park.

- Exit the park by taking a left onto SW Canby St. Turn right on SW 40th Ave., walk one block, then turn left onto SW Troy St., which you'll follow into the tiny Multnomah Village town center.

- When you reach SW 35th Ave., turn right. Cross over SW Capitol Hwy. and continue straight along SW 35th. Here on your left are a few cute shops and cafés, and on your right all the necessities: a pie shop and The Ship Tavern. The pie shop, Lovin Spoonful, is primarily a take-and-bake store, but there's also a coffee loft where you can sit down with a slice or a pastry. The Ship is an old Multnomah Village standby— a vaguely nautically themed dive with pool tables and sports on TV. The floor is usually covered in peanut shells, which gives the place a nice crunch. There's nothing even remotely fancy about The Ship, and it's not necessarily the place you want to go for food (most people just stick with the peanuts), but it's a great neighborhood bar all the same.

- Leaving The Ship, continue down SW 35th Ave. to SW Multnomah Blvd. and turn right. At the corner is John's Market, known far and wide for its vast selection of rare, imported, seasonal, and just top-notch bottled beer and wine (it claims the largest selection in Portland), as well as kegs of hard-to-find imported beer. There's also a good deli here.

- Where Multnomah meets SW Capitol Hwy. in an acute angle, turn right on Capitol to walk along the main commercial center of the village. For its size, Multnomah Village has a remarkably large number of good places in which to eat and drink— mostly the latter. On your right you'll find O'Connor's, whose brick building takes up three shopfronts. O'Connor's used to be in downtown Portland; it was founded in 1934, by Ed O'Connor of Butte, Montana. The original spot's dubious claim to fame is that, according to its website, it was one of the very last men-only bars in Portland. (These days, of course, we can all enjoy it.) A great rooftop deck is open all year.

- A couple of doors down is Annie Bloom's Books, established in 1978 and one of the coziest, most inviting independent bookshops in Portland. There's a store cat, of course, and the shop regularly hosts author readings.

- Also on this strip is the well-loved Fat City Cafe, a neighborhood diner serving greasy-spoon breakfasts in a kitsch-plastered space. The food might not be all that memorable, but the diner has a permanent place in local history, thanks to what has come to be known as the "Fat City Firing." In 1987, then-Mayor Bud Clark was sitting here having breakfast with his police chief when whatever conversation they were having ended in Clark's famous remark, "Read my lips: You're fired." Look for a sign over one of the booths commemorating the dismissal.

- Across the street is another great local dive, Renner's Grill, boasting one of the coolest neon signs in the area. It has everything you need in a dive bar: cheap, strong drinks; fried food; friendly locals; and not much else. Worth a stop!

- Continue along SW Capitol Hwy. and cross over SW 35th Ave. Walk several blocks (noting a stop for Bus 44 as you pass SW 33rd Ave.—you'll want to come back to this stop when you've finished the walk). When you reach SW 32nd Ave., you'll see on your left the Lucky Labrador Public House, which occupies a 1925 Masonic hall. (There are also Lucky Lab locations in Northwest Portland and on SE Hawthorne Blvd.) Feel free to cross the street and stop in for a pint, or continue straight along Capitol Hwy. for one more block.

- Duck right just briefly onto SW Canby St. to find Otto & Anita's Schnitzel Haus, an adorable Euro-style restaurant with a menu of various homemade schnitzels and other Bavarian specialties; it might be the only place around where you can satisfy your craving for dill-pickle soup.

- Return to the city center by hopping TriMet Bus 44 back to town; there's a stop at SW Capitol Hwy. and 33rd Ave., diagonally across the street from the Lucky Lab. (If you drove a car to the starting point and parked at Gabriel Park, simply retrace your steps and cut through the park to return to the parking lot.)

POINTS OF INTEREST (START TO FINISH)

Lovin Spoonful Pies lovinspoonfulpieshop.com, 7825 SW 35th Ave., 503-246-4533

The Ship Tavern 7827 SW 35th Ave., 503-244-7345

John's Market johnsmarketplace.com, 3535 SW Multnomah Blvd., 503-244-2617

O'Connor's oconnorsportland.com, 7850 SW Capitol Hwy., 503-244-1690

Annie Bloom's Books annieblooms.com, 7834 SW Capitol Hwy., 503-246-0053

Fat City Cafe 7820 SW Capitol Hwy., 503-245-5457

Renner's Grill rennersgrill.com, 7819 SW Capitol Hwy., 503-246-9097

Lucky Labrador Public House luckylab.com, 7675 SW Capitol Hwy., 503-244-2537

Otto & Anita's Schnitzel Haus ottoandanitas.com, 3025 SW Canby St., 503-452-1411

ROUTE SUMMARY

1. Start at the northeast corner of Gabriel Park.
2. At the fork, take the right-hand path.
3. At the baseball field, take the left-hand fork.
4. Turn left onto SW Canby St. to exit the park.
5. Turn right on SW 40th Ave.
6. Turn left on SW Troy St.
7. Turn right on SW 35th Ave.
8. Turn right on SW Multnomah Blvd.
9. Turn right on SW Capitol Hwy.
10. Duck right onto SW Canby St.

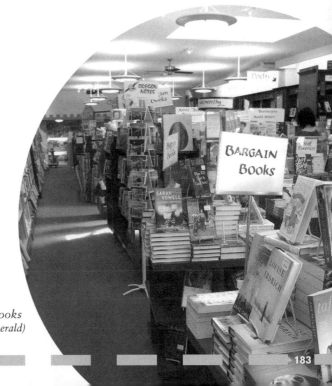

Annie Bloom's Books
(Photo courtesy of Paul Gerald)

Appendix 1: WALKS BY THEME

Park Life (Routes That Include Parks or Forests)

Downtown Park Blocks (Walk 2)
Goose Hollow (Walk 5)
Washington Park (Walk 6)
Forest Park (Walk 7)
Chapman School to Leif Erikson Drive
    (Walk 8)
Hawthorne Bridge to Steel Bridge (Walk 10)
Hawthorne Boulevard (Walk 14)
Stark-Belmont (Walk 15)
Kerns and Laurelhurst Park (Walk 17)
Fremont to Williams (Walk 21)
Historic Kenton (Walk 24)
St. Johns and Cathedral Park (Walk 25)
Columbia River Walk (Walk 26)
Lents (Walk 27)
Sellwood (Walk 29)

Eating and Drinking

Old Town and Chinatown (Walk 1)
Pearl District (Walk 3)
Northwest 21st and 23rd Avenues (Walk 4)

Industrial Southeast (Walk 12)
Division/Clinton, Ladd's Addition (Walk 13)
Hawthorne Boulevard (Walk 14)
Stark-Belmont (Walk 15)
Montavilla (Walk 16)
Kerns and Laurelhurst Park (Walk 17)
Irvington (Walk 18)
Hollywood (Walk 19)
Upper Sandy (Walk 20)
Fremont to Williams (Walk 21)
Mississippi to Killingsworth (Walk 22)
Alberta Arts District (Walk 23)
Multnomah Village (Walk 30)

History

Old Town and Chinatown (Walk 1)
Downtown Park Blocks (Walk 2)
Forest Park (Walk 7)
Reed College and Woodstock (Walk 28)

UP AND COMING (NEIGHBORHOODS IN FLUX)

Nicolai and Slabtown (Walk 9)
Tram to South Waterfront (Walk 11)
Industrial Southeast (Walk 12)
Montavilla (Walk 16)
Fremont to Williams (Walk 21)

RIVERS AND BRIDGES

Old Town and Chinatown (Walk 1)
Hawthorne Bridge to Steel Bridge (Walk 10)
Tram to South Waterfront (Walk 11)
Hawthorne Boulevard (Walk 14)
St. Johns and Cathedral Park (Walk 25)
Columbia River Walk (Walk 26)
Sellwood (Walk 29)

FARTHER AFIELD (WALKS THAT ARE SLIGHTLY OUT OF THE WAY)

Historic Kenton (Walk 24)
St. Johns and Cathedral Park (Walk 25)
Columbia River Walk (Walk 26)
Lents (Walk 27)
Multnomah Village (Walk 30)

Appendix 2: POINTS OF INTEREST

ENTERTAINMENT AND NIGHTLIFE

Academy Theater academytheaterpdx.com, 7818 SE Stark St., 503-252-0500 (Walk 16)

Acapulco's Gold 2608–10 NW Vaughn St., 503-220-0283 (Walk 8)

Alberta Rose Theatre albertarosetheatre.com, 3000 NE Alberta St., 503-719-6055 (Walk 23)

Avalon Theatre and Wunderland wunderlandgames.com/avalontheatre.asp, 3451 SE Belmont St., 503-238-1617 (Walk 15)

Backspace backspace.bz, 115 NW 5th Ave., 503-248-2900 (Walk 1)

Bagdad Theater & Pub mcmenamins.com/bagdad, 3702 SE Hawthorne Blvd., 503-467-7521 (Walk 14)

Bar of the Gods barofthegods.com, 4801 SE Hawthorne Blvd., 503-232-2037 (Walk 14)

Casa del Matador 1438 NW 23rd Ave., 503-228-2855 (Walk 4)

Cinema 21 cinema21.com, 616 NW 21st Ave., 503-223-4515 (Walk 4)

The CineMagic Theatre thecinemagictheater.com, 2021 SE Hawthorne Blvd., 503-231-7919 (Walk 14)

Clinton Street Theater cstpdx.com, 2522 SE Clinton St., 503-238-5588 (Walk 13)

Clinton Street Video 2501 SE Clinton St., 503-236-9030 (Walk 13)

Doug Fir Lounge dougfirlounge.com, 830 E. Burnside St., 503-231-9663 (Walk 12)

George's Dancin' Bare georgesdancinbare.com, 8440 N. Interstate Ave., 503-285-9073 (Walk 26)

Ground Kontrol groundkontrol.com, 511 NW Couch St., 503-796-9364 (Walk 1)

Hanigan's Tavern (a.k.a. The Vern) 2622 SE Belmont St., 503-233-7851 (Walk 15)

Hawthorne Theatre hawthornetheatre.com, 1507 SE 39th Ave., 503-233-7100 (Walk 14)

Hollywood Theatre hollywoodtheatre.org, 4122 NE Sandy Blvd., 503-493-1128 (Walk 19)

The Know theknowbar.com, 2026 NE Alberta St., 503-473-8729 (Walk 23)

Laurelhurst Theater laurelhursttheater.com, 2735 E. Burnside St., 503-232-5511 (Walk 17)

Mississippi Studios and Bar Bar mississippistudios.com, 3939 N. Mississippi Ave., 503-288-3895 (Walk 22)

Moreland Theater morelandtheater.com, 6712 SE Milwaukie Ave., 503-236-5257 (Walk 29)

Movie Madness moviemadnessvideo.com, 4320 SE Belmont St., 503-234-4363 (Walk 15)

New Copper Penny 5932 SE 92nd Ave., 503-777-1415 (Walk 27)

Pirate's Cove piratescoveportland.com, 7417 NE Sandy Blvd., 503-287-8900 (Walk 20)

Portland Tub and Tan tubandtan.com, 8028 SE Stark St., 503-261-1180 (Walk 16)

Roseway Theater rosewaytheater.com, 7229 NE Sandy Blvd., 503-282-2898 (Walk 20)

St. Johns Theater & Pub mcmenamins.com/stjohns, 8203 N. Ivanhoe St., 503-283-8520 (Walk 25)

The Sandy Hut sandyhut.com, 1430 NE Sandy Blvd., 503-235-7972 (Walk 17)

Slabtown slabtownbar.net, 1033 NW 16th Ave., 971-229-1455 (Walk 9)

Space Room Lounge spaceroomlounge.com, 4800 SE Hawthorne Blvd., 503-235-6957 (Walk 14)

White Eagle mcmenamins.com/whiteeaglesaloon, 836 N. Russell St., 503-282-6810 (Walk 22)

Wishing Well 8800 N. Lombard St., 503-286-4434 (Walk 25)

The World Famous Kenton Club kentonclub.com, 2025 N. Kilpatrick St., 503-285-3718 (Walk 24)

FOOD aND DrINK

21st Avenue Bar & Grill 21stbarandgrill.com, 721 NW 21st Ave., 503-222-4121 (Walk 4)

Albina Press 5012 SE Hawthorne Blvd., 503-282-5214 (Walk 14)

Amnesia Brewing amnesiabrews.com, 832 N. Beech St., 503-281-7708 (Walk 22)

Annie's Donuts 3449 NE 72nd Ave., 503-284-2752 (Walk 20)

APEX apexbar.com, 1216 SE Division St., 503-273-9227 (Walk 13)

Ararat Bakery 5716 SE 92nd Ave., 503-235-5526 (Walk 27)

Bambuza Vietnam Bistro bambuza.com, 3682 SW Bond Ave., 503-206-6330 (Walk 11)

Barista baristapdx.com, 539 NW 13th Ave. (Walk 3)

Belmont Station belmont-station.com, 4500 SE Stark St., 503-232-8538 (Walk 15)

Bipartisan Cafe bipartisancafe.com, 7901 SE Stark St., 503-253-1051 (Walk 16)

Le Bistro Montage montageportland.com, 301 SE Morrison St., 503-234-1324 (Walk 12)

Breken Kitchen brekenkitchen.com, 1800 NW 16th Ave., 503-841-6359 (Walk 9)

BridgePort Brew Pub bridgeportbrew.com, 1313 NW Marshall St., 503-241-3612 (Walk 9)

The Bye and Bye thebyeandbye.com, 1011 NE Alberta St., 503-281-0537

Caldera Public House calderapublichouse.com, 6031 SE Stark St., 503-233-8242 (Walk 15)

Candlelight Restaurant & Lounge 7334 NE Glisan St., 503-253-9738 (Walk 16)

Castagna castagnarestaurant.com, 1752 SE Hawthorne Blvd., 503-231-7373

Chapel Pub mcmenamins.com/chapel, 430 N. Killingsworth St., 503-286-0372 (Walk 22)

Cheese Bar cheese-bar.com, 6031 SE Belmont St., 503-222-6014 (Walk 15)

Club 21 2035 NE Glisan St., 503-235-5690 (Walk 17)

Clyde's Prime Rib clydesprimerib.com, 5474 NE Sandy Blvd., 503-281-9200 (Walk 20)

The Country Cat thecountrycat.net, 7937 SE Stark St., 503-408-1414 (Walk 16)

Daily Cafe at the Tram dailycafe.net, 3355 SW Bond Ave., 503-224-9691 (Walk 11)

Delta Cafe deltacafepdx.com, 4607 SE Woodstock Blvd., 503-771-3101 (Walk 28)

Dots Cafe 2521 SE Clinton St., 503-235-0203 (Walk 13)

Driftwood Room graciesdining.com/driftwood.html, 729 SW 15th Ave., 503-222-2171 (Walk 5)

East Side Deli pdxdeli.com, 4626 SE Hawthorne Blvd., 503-236-7313 (Walk 14)

Escape From New York Pizza efnypizza.net, 622 NW 23rd Ave., 503-227-5423 (Walk 4)

Fairley's Pharmacy 7206 NE Sandy Blvd., 503-284-1159 (Walk 20)

Fat City Cafe 7820 SW Capitol Hwy., 503-245-5457 (Walk 30)

Fifteenth Avenue Hophouse oregonhophouse.com, 1517 NE Brazee St., 971-266-8392 (Walk 18)

Fifth Quadrant lompocbrewing.com, 3901 N. Williams Ave., 503-288-3996 (Walk 21)

Fleur de Lis fleurdelisbakery.com, 3930 NE Hancock St., 503-459-4887 (Walk 19)

Flying Pie Pizzeria flying-pie.com, 7804 SE Stark St., 503-254-2016 (Walk 16)

The Florida Room 435 N. Killingsworth St., 503-287-5658 (Walk 22)

Gino's ginossellwood.com, 8051 SE 13th Ave., 503-233-4613 (Walk 29)

Goose Hollow Inn goosehollowinn.com, 1927 SW Jefferson St., 503-228-7010 (Walk 5)

Grand Central Bakery grandcentralbakery.com, 2230 SE Hawthorne Blvd., 503-445-1600 (Walk 14)

The Gypsy cegportland.com/gypsy, 625 NW 21st Ave., 503-796-1859 (Walk 4)

Hair of the Dog Brewing Company hairofthedog.com, 61 SE Water Ave., 503-232-6585 (Walk 12)

Heart Roasters heartroasters.com, 2211 E. Burnside St., 503-206-6602 (Walk 17)

Hollywood Burger Bar hollywoodburgerbar.com, 4211 NE Sandy Blvd., 503-288-6422 (Walk 19)

Hopworks BikeBar hopworksbeer.com, 3947 N. Williams Ave., 503-287-6258 (Walk 21)

Horse Brass Pub horsebrass.com, 4534 SE Belmont St., 503-232-2202 (Walk 15)

Hotlips hotlipspizza.com, NW 10th Ave. and Irving St., 503-595-2342 (Walk 3)

Kenny & Zuke's Bagelworks kzbagelworks.com, 2376 NW Thurman St., 503-954-1737 (Walk 8)

La Sirenita 2817 NE Alberta St., 503-335-8283 (Walk 23)

Laurelwood Public House laurelwoodbrewpub.com, 5115 NE Sandy Blvd., 503-282-0622 (Walk 19)

Le Happy lehappy.com, 1011 NW 16th Ave., 503-226-1258 (Walk 9)

Los Gorditos losgorditospdx.com, 1212 SE Division St., 503-445-6289 (Walk 13)

Lovin Spoonful Pies lovinspoonfulpieshop.com, 7825 SW 35th Ave., 503-246-4533 (Walk 30)

Low Brow Lounge 1036 NW Hoyt St., 503-226-0200 (Walk 3)

Lucky Labrador Beer Hall luckylab.com, 1945 NW Quimby St., 503-517-4352 (Walk 9)

Lucky Labrador Public House luckylab.com, 7675 SW Capitol Hwy., 503-244-2537 (Walk 30)

Lutz Tavern 4639 SE Woodstock Blvd., 503-774-0353 (Walk 28)

Milepost 5 milepost5.net, 850 NE 81st Ave. (Walk 16)

The Moon and Sixpence 2014 NE 42nd Ave., 503-288-7802 (Walk 19)

Muu-Muu's muumuus.net, 612 NW 21st Ave., 503-223-8196 (Walk 4)

Night Light Lounge nightlightlounge.net, 2100 SE Clinton St., 503-731-6500 (Walk 13)

Occidental Brewing Co. occidentalbrewing.com, 6635 N. Baltimore Ave., 503-719-7102 (Walk 25)

O'Connor's oconnorsportland.com, 7850 SW Capitol Hwy., 503-244-1690 (Walk 30)

Olympic Provisions olympicprovisions.com, 1632 NW Thurman St., 503-894-8136 (Walk 9)

Otto & Anita's Schnitzel Haus ottoandanitas.com, 3025 SW Canby St., 503-452-1411 (Walk 30)

Oui Presse oui-presse.com, 1740 SE Hawthorne Blvd., 503-384-2160 (Walk 14)

Over and Out/The Observatory theobservatorypdx.com/overandoutbar.php, 410 SE 81st Ave., 503-445-6284 (Walk 16)

Palio Dessert & Espresso House palio-in-ladds.com, 1996 SE Ladd Ave., 503-232-9412 (Walk 13)

Pambiche pambiche.com, 2811 NE Glisan St., 503-233-0511 (Walk 17)

Papa Haydn papahaydn.com, 5829 SE Milwaukie Ave., 503-232-9440 (Walk 29)

Le Pigeon lepigeon.com, 738 E. Burnside St., 503-546-8796 (Walk 12)

Pok Pok pokpokpdx.com, 3226 SE Division St., 503-232-1387 (Walk 13)

Pope House Bourbon Lounge popehouselounge.com, 2075 NW Glisan St., 503-222-1056 (Walk 4)

¿Por Qué No? porquenotacos.com, 4635 SE Hawthorne Blvd., 503-954-3138 (Walk 14)

Posies Bakery & Cafe posiescafe.com, 8208 N. Denver Ave., 503-289-1319 (Walk 24)

Produce Row Café producerowcafe.com, 204 SE Oak St., 503-232-8355 (Walk 12)

Renner's Grill rennersgrill.com, 7819 SW Capitol Hwy., 503-246-9097 (Walk 30)

Rilassi Coffee House & Tea rilassicoffeehouse.com, 3580 SW River Pkwy., 503-467-7532 (Walk 11)

RingSide Steakhouse ringsidesteakhouse.com, 2165 W. Burnside St., 503-223-1513 (Walk 4)

Ristretto Roasters ristrettoroasters.com, 2181 NW Nicolai St., 503-227-2866 (Walk 9)

Ristretto Roasters ristrettoroasters.com, 3520 NE 42nd Ave., 503-284-6767 (Walk 21)

St. Honoré Bakery sainthonorebakery.com, 2335 NW Thurman St., 503-445-4342 (Walk 8)

Salt & Straw saltandstraw.com, 2035 NE Alberta St., 503-208-3867 (Walk 23)

Sapphire Hotel thesapphirehotel.com, 5008 SE Hawthorne Blvd., 503-232-6333 (Walk 14)

See See Motor Coffee Co. seeseemotorcycles.com, 1642 NE Sandy Blvd., 503-894-9566 (Walk 17)

The Ship Tavern 7827 SW 35th Ave., 503-244-7345 (Walk 30)

Signal Station Pizza signalstationpizza.com, 8302 N. Lombard St., 503-286-2257 (Walk 25)

TaborSpace taborspace.org, 5441 SE Belmont St., 503-238-3904 (Walk 15)

Tasty n Sons tastynsons.com, 3808 N. Williams Ave., 503-621-1400 (Walk 21)

Vendetta vendettapdx.com, 4306 N. Williams Ave., 503-288-1085 (Walk 21)

Victory Bar thevictorybar.com, 3652 SE Division St., 503-236-8755 (Walk 13)

Vita Cafe vita-cafe.com, 3023 NE Alberta St., 503-335-8233 (Walk 23)

Voodoo Doughnut voodoodoughnut.com, 22 SW 3rd Ave., 503-241-4704 (Walk 1)

Voodoo Doughnut Too voodoodoughnut.com, 1501 NE Davis St., 503-235-2666 (Walk 17)

Water Avenue Coffee wateravenuecoffee.com, 1028 SE Water Ave., 503-808-7083 (Walk 12)

Widmer Brothers Brewing Company widmerbrothers.com/brewery, 929 N. Russell St., 503-281-2437 (Walk 22)

Ya Hala Lebanese Restaurant yahalarestaurant.com, 8005 SE Stark St., 503-256-4484 (Walk 16)

Yukon Tavern 5819 SE Milwaukie Ave., 503-235-6352 (Walk 29)

MUSEUMS

24 Hour Church of Elvis 24hourchurchofelvis.com, 408 NW Couch St. (Walk 1)

Freakybuttrue Peculiarium peculiarium.com, 2234 NW Thurman St. (Walk 9)

The Hat Museum thehatmuseum.com, 1928 SE Ladd Ave., 503-232-0433 (Walk 13)

Laura Russo Gallery laurarusso.com, 805 NW 21st Ave., 503-226-2754 (Walk 4)

Museum of Contemporary Craft museumofcontemporarycraft.org, 724 NW Davis St., 503-223-2654 (Walk 3)

Oregon Museum of Science and Industry omsi.edu, 1945 SE Water Ave., 503-797-4640 (Walk 12)

The Oregon Historical Society ohs.org, 1200 SW Park Ave., 503-222-1741 (Walk 2)

Oregon Maritime Museum oregonmaritimemuseum.org, 115 SW Ash St., 503-224-7724 (Walk 10)

Pittock Mansion pittockmansion.org, 3229 NW Pittock Dr., 503-823-3623 (Walk 7)

Portland Art Museum pam.org, 1219 SW Park Ave., 503-226-2811 (Walk 2)

Portland Children's Museum portlandcm.org, 4015 SW Canyon Rd., 503-223-6500 (Walk 6)

Stark's Vacuum Museum starks.com, 107 NE Grand Ave., 800-230-4101 (Walk 12)

World Forestry Center worldforestry.org, 4033 SW Canyon Rd., 503-228-1367 (Walk 6)

NOTABLE BUILDINGS

Alberta Substation 2703 NE Alberta St. (Walk 23)

Ecotrust Building 721 NW 9th Ave. (Walk 3)

Fire Station 28 5540 NE Sandy Blvd. (Walk 20)

Jeld-Wen Field jeld-wenfield.com, SE Morrison St. and 18th Ave. (Hike 5)

Keana's Candyland keanascandyland.net, 5314 SE Milwaukie Ave., 503-719-5131 (Walk 29)

Lion and the Rose Victorian Bed & Breakfast lionrose.com, 1810 NE 15th Ave., 503-287-9245 (Walk 18)

Miao Fa Temple miaofatemple.com, 1722 SE Madison St., 503-239-5678 (Walk 14)

North Portland Library multcolib.org, 512 N. Killingsworth St., 503-988-5394 (Walk 22)

Oaks Pioneer Church oakspioneerchurch.org, 455 SE Spokane St. (Walk 29)

Olympic Mills Commerce Center 107 SE Washington St. (Walk 12)

Portland's White House portlandswhitehouse.com, 1914 NE 22nd Ave., 503-287-7131 (Walk 18)

Portland Building 1120 SW 5th Ave. (Walk 2)

Sellwood-Moreland Library multcolib.org, 7860 SE 13th Ave., 503-988-5398 (Walk 29)

St. Andrew Catholic Church standrewchurch.com, 806 NE Alberta St., 503-281-4429 (Walk 23)

Wieden + Kennedy wk.com, 224 NW 13th Ave., 503-937-7000 (Walk 3)

Wilhelm's Portland Memorial Funeral Home 6705 SE 14th Ave. (Walk 29)

Parks and Gardens

Burnside Skatepark East side of Burnside Bridge (Walk 12)

Crystal Springs Rhododendron Garden rhodies.org, SE 28th Ave. and Woodstock Blvd., 503-771-8386 (Walk 28)

The Grotto thegrotto.org, NE 85th Ave. and Sandy Blvd., 503-254-7371 (Walk 20)

Hoyt Arboretum hoytarboretum.org, 4000 SW Fairview Blvd., 503-865-8733 (Walk 6)

International Rose Test Garden tinyurl.com/rosetestgarden, 850 SW Rose Garden Way, 503-823-3636 (Walk 6)

Japanese Garden japanesegarden.com, 611 SW Kingston Ave., 503-223-1321 (Walk 6)

Kenton Park 8417 N. Brandon Ave. (Walk 24)

Lan Su Chinese Garden portlandchinesegarden.org, 239 NW Everett St., 503-228-8131 (Walk 1)

Lone Fir Pioneer Cemetery friendsoflonefircemetery.org, SE 26th Ave. between Stark and Morrison Sts. (Walk 15)

Marquam Nature Park fmnp.org, SW Sam Jackson Park Rd. and SW Marquam St. (Walk 11)

Oaks Amusement Park oakspark.com, 7805 SE Oaks Park Way, 503-233-5777 (Walk 29)

Oaks Bottom Wildlife Refuge tinyurl.com/oaksbottom, SE Milwaukie Ave. and Mitchell St. (Walk 29)

Oregon Zoo oregonzoo.org, 4001 SW Canyon Rd., 503-226-1561 (Walk 6)

Portland International Raceway portlandraceway.com, 1940 N. Victory Blvd. (Walk 26)

Rose City Cemetery 5625 NE Fremont St. (Walk 21)

Smith and Bybee Wetlands Natural Area 5300 N. Marine Dr. (Walk 26)

Shopping

3 Monkeys 811 NW 23rd Ave., 503-222-5160 (Walk 4)

Annie Bloom's Books annieblooms.com, 7834 SW Capitol Hwy., 503-246-0053 (Walk 30)

Bridge City Comics bridgecitycomics.com, 3725 N. Mississippi Ave., 503-282-5484 (Walk 22)

Broadway Books broadwaybooks.net, 1714 NE Broadway, 503-284-1726 (Walk 18)

Clear Creek Distillery clearcreekdistillery.com, 2389 NW Wilson St., 503-248-9470 (Walk 9)

Excalibur Books & Comics excaliburcomics.net, 2444 SE Hawthorne Blvd., 503-231-7351 (Walk 14)

Fat Tire Farm fattirefarm.com, 2714 NW Thurman St., 503-222-3276 (Walk 8)

Floating World Comics floatingworldcomics.com, 400 NW Couch St., 503-241-0227 (Walk 1)

Food Front Cooperative Grocery foodfront.coop, 2375 NW Thurman St., 503-222-5658 (Walk 8)

Green Bean Books greenbeanbookspdx.com, 1600 NE Alberta St., 503-954-2354 (Walk 23)

Hawthorne Boulevard Books 3129 SE Hawthorne Blvd., 503-236-3211 (Walk 14)

Hippo Hardware hippohardware.com, 1040 E. Burnside St., 503-231-1444 (Walk 12)

Hollywood Farmers Market hollywoodfarmersmarket.org, NE Hancock St. between 44th and 45th Aves. (Walk 19)

In Other Words inotherwords.org, 14 NE Killingsworth St., 503-232-6003 (Walk 22)

John's Market johnsmarketplace.com, 3535 SW Multnomah Blvd., 503-244-2617 (Walk 30)

Kenton Antiques kentonantiquespdx.com, 8112 N. Denver Ave., 503-490-8855 (Walk 24)

Langlitz Leathers langlitz.com, 2443 SE Division St., 503-235-0959 (Walk 13)

Lents International Farmers Market lentsfarmersmarket.org, SE 92nd and Foster Rd. (Walk 27)

Lloyd Center lloydcenter.com, 2201 Lloyd Center, 503-282-2511 (Walk 18)

Monograph Bookwerks monographbookwerks.com, 5005 NE 27th Ave., 503-284-5005 (Walk 23)

Montavilla Farmers Market montavillamarket.org, 7600 block of SE Stark St. (Walk 16)

Murder by the Book mbtb.com, 3210 SE Hawthorne Blvd., 503-232-9995 (Walk 14)

Music Millennium musicmillennium.com, 3158 E. Burnside St., 503-231-8926 (Walk 17)

New Renaissance Bookshop newrenbooks.com, 1338 NW 23rd Ave., 503-224-4929 (Walk 4)

Oblation Papers & Press oblationpapers.com, 516 NW 12th Ave., 503-223-1093 (Walk 3)

Paxton Gate paxtongatepdx.com, 4204 N. Mississippi Ave., 503-719-4508 (Walk 22)

Portland Preparedness Center getreadyportland.com, 7202 NE Glisan St., 503-252-2525 (Walk 16)

Powell's City of Books powells.com, 1005 W. Burnside St., 503-228-4651 (Walk 3)

Powell's Books on Hawthorne powells.com, 3723 SE Hawthorne Blvd., 503-228-4651 (Walk 14)

The Raven ravenantiques.com, 7927 SE 13th Ave., 503-233-8075 (Walk 29)

The ReBuilding Center rebuildingcenter.org, 3625 N. Mississippi Ave., 503-331-1877 (Walk 22)

Record Room recordroompdx.com, 8 NE Killingsworth St., 971-544-7685 (Walk 22)

Rich's Cigar Store richscigar.com, 706 NW 23rd Ave., 503-227-6907 (Walk 4)

Salvage Works, Boys Fort, Solabee Flowers salvageworkspdx.com, 2030 N. Willis Blvd., 503-285-2555 (Walk 24)

Schoolhouse Electric & Supply Co. schoolhouseelectric.com, 2181 NW Nicolai St., 503-230-7113 (Walk 9)

Second Glance Books secondglancebooks.com, 4500 NE Sandy Blvd., 503-249-0344 (Walk 19)

Sheridan Fruit Company sheridanfruit.com, 409 SE Martin Luther King Jr. Blvd., 503-236-2114 (Walk 12)

Stars Antiques Mall starsantique.com, 7027 SE Milwaukie Ave., 503-239-0346 (Walk 29)

Sunlan Lighting sunlanlighting.com, 3901 N. Mississippi Ave., 503-281-0453 (Walk 22)

Urban Farm Store urbanfarmstore.com, 2100 SE Belmont St., 503-234-7733 (Walk 15)

INFOrMaTION/MISCeLLaNeOUS

Friendly House friendlyhouseinc.org, 1737 NW 26th Ave., 503-228-4391 (Walk 8)

Hawthorne Portland Hostel portlandhostel.org, 3031 SE Hawthorne Blvd., 503-236-3380 (Walk 14)

Montavilla Community Center 8219 NE Glisan St., 503-823-4101 (Walk 16)

North Portland Tool Library northportlandtoollibrary.org, 2209 N. Schofield St., 503-823-0209 (Walk 24)

Portland Tub and Tan tubandtan.com, 8028 SE Stark St., 503-261-1180

Reed College reed.edu (Walk 28)

Tin House **Magazine** tinhouse.com, 2617 NW Thurman St. (Walk 8)

Travel Portland Visitor Information Center travelportland.com, 701 SW 6th Ave., 503-275-8355 (Walk 2)

Woodstock Community Center 5905 SE 43rd Ave., 503-823-3633 (Walk 28)

INDEX

about the author

BECKY OHLSEN has lived in Portland for the past 15 or so years. She's a freelance writer and editor who has contributed to a variety of publications, including the Pulitzer-winning newsweekly *Willamette Week, The Oregonian, Portland Monthly*, and Lonely Planet,

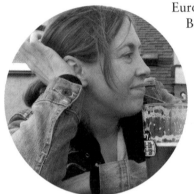

for which she has written several guidebooks about Scandinavian Europe and the Pacific Northwest. When she isn't out walking, Becky usually gets around by motorcycle; she's a member of the Sang-Froid Riding Club, and she served on the City of Portland's volunteer Motorcycles & Scooters Citizen Advisory Committee. She also occasionally reviews movies on the KQAC All Classical radio station's podcast *On the Aisle*. Becky has a master's degree in journalism from New York University's Cultural Reporting and Criticism (CRC) program and currently works as a legal editor at a downtown-Portland law firm.

Photo courtesy of Rob Seamans